AF333044

HEPATITIS C VIRUS: EPIDEMIOLOGY, PATHOGENESIS AND TREATMENT

VIROLOGY RESEARCH PROGRESS

Additional books in this series can be found on Nova's website
under the Series tab.

Additional E-books in this series can be found on Nova's website
under the E-book tab.

HEPATOLOGY RESEARCH AND CLINICAL DEVELOPMENTS

Additional books in this series can be found on Nova's website
under the Series tab.

Additional E-books in this series can be found on Nova's website
under the E-book tab.

VIROLOGY RESEARCH PROGRESS

HEPATITIS C VIRUS: EPIDEMIOLOGY, PATHOGENESIS AND TREATMENT

ALVARO PEREZ GONZALES

AND

ANGEL ALONSO VERRACRUZ

EDITORS

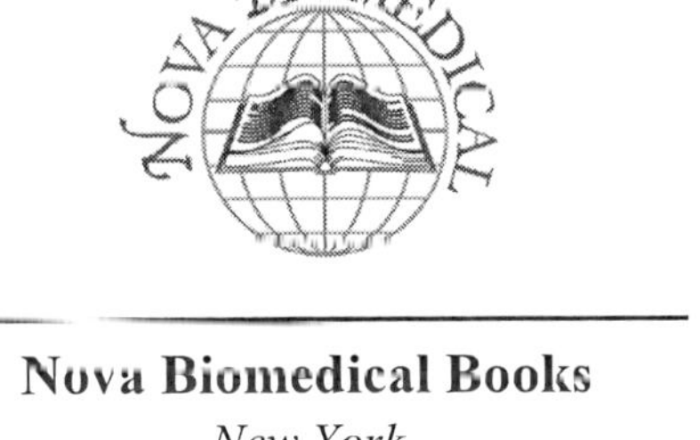

Nova Biomedical Books

New York

Library of Congress Cataloging-in-Publication Data

ISBN 978-1-61942-674-0

Library of Congress Control Number: 2011946019

Published by Nova Science Publishers, Inc. † New York

Contents

Preface

Chronic Hepatitis C virus (HCV) infection is a serious condition affecting over 180 million people worldwide. The virus infects the liver and while it is estimated that 20% of those infected clear the virus spontaneously, the virus persists in the majority of individuals leading to liver fibrosis, cirrhosis, and hepatocellular carcinoma. This book presents topical research in the study of the epidemiology, pathogenesis and treatment of Hepatitic C Virus including: genome-wide association studies regarding HCV infection; hepatic and blood dendritic cell subsets in patients with chronic HCV; bone metabolism disorders in HCV infection; Socs1 involvement in liver damage during HCV infection; asymptomatic low-level HCV persistence; and HCV infection as the leading cause of liver disease in renal transplant recipients.

Chapter I - Existing lines of evidence have highlighted the beginning of a genomic era for the management of hepatitis C virus (HCV) infection. Several research groups from different countries using the approaches of genome-wide association studies (GWAS) simultaneously identified the polymorphism of IL28B gene as an important predictor of therapeutic response for chronic hepatitis C (CHC) patients receiving interferon-based treatment in 2009. Moreover, they also found that host genetic variations near IL28B gene also play an important role in the spontaneous clearance of HCV. On the other hand, inosine triphosphate pyrophosphatase (ITPA) gene variants are reported to affect ribavirin-induced anemia and therapeutic outcomes in CHC patients. In this article, recent advances in genome-wide association studies regarding HCV infection, and their impacts on current management of CHC patients will be reviewed. In addition, the clinical usefulness of genomic variations on the addition of direct antiviral agents (DAAs) to current standard of care will be discussed.

Chapter II – Dendritic cells (DCs) are key mediators of innate anti-viral immunity being important detectors of viral infection and potent producers of Type I interferons (IFNs), IFN-α and IFN-β, as well as Type III IFNs, the IFN-λs. Successful adaptive anti-viral immunity also relies on the antigen presenting capacity of DCs and their production of cytokines that influence T cell polarisation. Defective immunity in patients with chronic Hepatitis C virus (HCV) infection has been proposed to be due to DC dysfunction which may also explain the poor success in generating therapeutic or preventative vaccination strategies for HCV infection. However, the many studies which have examined DC frequency and function in HCV patients to date have yielded conflicting results and the topic remains controversial. This may be because there are heterogeneous DC populations including myeloid and plasmacytoid lineages with various subsets of DCs having functional specialisations and different tissue localisation. In addition, little is known about the DC subtypes that predominate in human liver, the primary site of HCV replication, with the major studies being carried out in mice due to difficulty in obtaining human liver tissue and isolating DCs. Here the authors review the literature on DC subsets from HCV-infected blood and liver and make suggestions for future studies in this area that might lead to an improved understanding of HCV immunity and provide us with additional therapeutic targets.

Chapter III - Hepatic osteodystrophy (HO) is an important complication of chronic liver disease with an estimated prevalence ranging between 10 and 50%. Osteopenia and osteoporosis associated to liver disease result in increased morbidity due to bone fractures, chronic pain and immobility. Cholestasis liver diseases such as primary biliary cirrhosis are the conditions causing HO more frequently, but other liver diseases like haemochromatosis, alcoholic liver disease and chronic viral hepatitis are also responsible of bone impairment.

Loss of bone mineral density (BMD) occurs in patients with chronic hepatitis C virus (HCV) infection, being more frequent and severe in HCV cirrhosis with a prevalence of 20%-53%. The aim of this chapter is to summarize some practical issues regarding this topic and to provide a review about the main pathophysiological and therapeutic aspects.

Althought little is known about pathogenesis of HO in chronic HCV infection, it seems to be multifactorial. Bone loss occurs as a result of increased bone turnover and/or remodelling imbalance, being the latter caused by a reduced formation, an increased resorption or a combination of both. Vitamin D metabolism is impaired in the presence of severe HCV disease, and deficiency of this vitamin may cause hyperparathyroidism, increased bone turnover and accelerated loss of BMD. Disregulation of RANKL/OPG system, activated by cytokines involved in the pathogenesis of chronic liver disease (IL-1, IL-6, TNFα), is a defined mechanism for HO in HCV infection. Genetic factors such as polymorphisms of vitamin D receptor gene, collagen type Iα1 gene and the insulin growth factor-1 (IGF-1) gene have also been investigated and proposed to play a role in the pathogenesis of bone disease.

General management of osteopenia and osteoporosis in chronic HCV infection includes a prompt evaluation and an early diagnosis of osteoporosis using dual-energy X-ray absorptiometry (DXA). Application of therapy must consider general measures (correction of reversible risk factors, calcium intake and supplementation) and specific treatment for osteoporosis. Bisphosphonates are antiresorptive drugs that can improve BMD in other chronic liver disease, but only limited data are available for osteoporosis in HCV infection. Likewise, little is known about the effect of antiviral agents against HCV on BMD and their potential benefit on bone impairment. Orthotopic liver transplantation is followed by a transient BMD loss in the early months, but in the long term post-transplant there is a positive effect and a recovery of bone density.

Osteopenia and osteoporosis are common complications in chronic HCV infection, affecting both cirrhotic and non-cirrhotic individuals. The underlying mechanisms are not thoroughly understood. Thus, physiopathological bases of HO secondary to HCV should be clearly established in order to define specific treatments aimed at preventing and altering its clinical evolution.

Chapter IV - Hepatitis C virus (HCV) is a public health concern worldwide and a major cause of hepatic cirrhosis and hepatocellular carcinoma (HCC). Current therapy for HCV infection is the administration of pegylated-interferon-alpha (IFN-α) plus ribavirin; however, ~50% of treated patients do not respond to interferon therapy and, thus, are not able to clear virus infection. IFN-α plays a pivotal role in the response against viral infections, acting through its specific cell receptors that activate the JAK-STAT signaling pathway and inducing the expression of hundreds of genes that code for proteins with antiviral functions. The antiviral activity generated by interferon is negatively controlled by several proteins, among them the suppressor of cytokine signaling 1 (SOCS1), which is a negative regulator of the JAK STAT signaling pathway induced by different cytokines (IFNα/β, IFNγ, IL-6 and IL-4). *Socs1* deficiency is associated with chronic liver alterations. Diploid knockout mice (SOCS1$^{-/-}$) presented fatty degeneration and hepatic necrosis, whereas haploid elimination (SOCS1$^{-/+}$) increased progression to hepatic fibrosis. In addition, silencing of *socs1* gene by methylation induced a permanent activation of the JAK-STAT pathway in HCC cell lines, suggesting that *socs1* is a tumor suppressor. In this chapter the authors review the participation of *socs1* in several molecular mechanisms involved in liver damage during HCV infection.

Chapter V - The existence of low-level hepatitis C virus (HCV) infection, termed as occult HCV infection (OCI) has been uncovered in this laboratory by applying assays with enhanced sensitivity and by testing patients' samples acquired from different compartments where the virus naturally occurs. Subsequent works conducted by us and others identified virological and immunological characteristics of OCI, and pointed out to potential pathological outcomes of this form of HCV infection. Occult HCV infection can persist in the presence of antibodies against HCV (anti-HCV) and normal liver enzymes for years after spontaneous or interferon alpha-ribavirin (IFN/RBV) therapy-induced resolution of hepatitis C. In addition to this residual or secondary occult infection, a low-level HCV infection of unknown etiology in individuals negative for anti-HCV antibodies with moderately elevated liver function enzymes has been described. This review will highlight works which led to the identification of OCI, outline known properties of the infection, present principles of OCI identification and factors influencing its detection, and summarize our current understanding of the documented and expected pathological consequences of OCI.

Chapter VI - HCV infection is the leading cause of liver disease in renal transplant (RTx) recipients. Despite its high frequency, the impact of immunosuppression on the evolution of the disease remains unclear while histopathological changes have not been thoroughly investigated.

Data referring to patients survival and hepatitis progression are still controversial. According to some reports, chronic hepatitis C (CHC) runs a rather benign course after transplantation showing a short-term survival similar to non-infected patients without significant difference in the severity of liver disease between hemodialysis and transplant patients. On the contrary, other studies demonstrated an adverse clinical outcome, especially after long-term follow-up. Although prognostic factors have not yet been precisely defined, duration of hepatitis and the severity of pre-existing liver disease seem to influence disease progression. Moreover, some data suggest that time of acquisition of HCV infection in relation to transplantation may present a prognostic parameter playing a significant role in hepatitis evolution. The majority of RTx recipients are infected with HCV while being on hemodialysis. A small number of patients acquire the infection shortly before, rarely during transplantation, and occasionally in the post-transplant period. There are indications that patients showing a milder clinical course were contaminated before transplantation and during the time period spent on hemodialysis. On the contrary, patients infected close to or after transplantation display an adverse hepatitis outcome.

Histologically, HCV infection presents as conventional acute and chronic hepatitis and rarely as fibrosing cholestatic hepatitis (FCH) and interlobular bile duct damage and loss. Acute hepatitis is generally mild. Chronic hepatitis is minimal or mild and only exceptionally of moderate severity. FCH and interlobular bile duct damage and loss occur mostly during the early and late post-transplant period, respectively. Liver cell apoptosis seems to be an important factor in liver injury closely linked to high viral load. The direct pathogenetic role of HCV is further supported by the association of both cholestatic syndromes and an adverse hepatitis evolution with high viremia levels.

Conclusively, time point of infection seems to be of major prognostic significance rendering immunosuppression as a crucial prognostic factor in the evolvement of hepatitis in patients that are infected at the time or after transplantation. The histological range includes besides conventional acute and chronic hepatitis, cholestatic diseases such as FCH and bile duct damage and loss. High viral load seems to play an important role in the pathogenesis, rendering an early reduction of the immunosuppressive therapy mandatory.

Chapter VII - It is well known that chronic hepatitis C virus (HCV) infection is the main cause of liver cirrhosis and hepatocellular carcinoma (HCC). In terms of the underlying mechanisms, many experimental and clinical studies have suggested that insulin resistance, oxidative stress, or subsequent abnormalglucose metabolism caused by obesity or HCV itself might play important roles in the progression of liver fibrosis and carcinogenesis. In this chapter, the authors discuss the associations between metabolic factors and the clinical course of HCV-infected patients.

In: Hepatitis C Virus
Editors: A. P. Gonzales et al.

ISBN 978-1-61942-674-0
© 2012 Nova Science Publishers, Inc.

Chapter I

Management of Hepatitis C Virus Infection in the Genomic Era

Ching-Sheng Hsu[1] and Jia-Horng Kao[2-5]*

[1]Division of Gastroenterology, Department of Internal Medicine,
Buddhist Tzu Chi General Hospital, Taipei Branch, and School of
Medicine, Tzu Chi University, Hualien, Taiwan
[2]Graduate Institute of Clinical Medicine
[3]Department of Internal Medicine
[4]Department of Medical Research
[5]Hepatitis Research Center, National Taiwan University
College of Medicine and National Taiwan University Hospital,
Taipei, Taiwan

ABSTRACT

Existing lines of evidence have highlighted the beginning of a
genomic era for the management of hepatitis C virus (HCV) infection.
Several research groups from different countries using the approaches of
genome-wide association studies (GWAS) simultaneously identified the

* Corresponding author: Dr. Jia-Horng Kao, Director and Distinguished Professor, Graduate
Institute of Clinical Medicine, National Taiwan University College of Medicine 7 Chung-
Shan South Road, Taipei 10002, Taiwan. Tel.: 886-2-23123456 ext 67307. Fax: 886-2-
23825962. E-mail: kaojh@ntu.edu.tw

polymorphism of IL28B gene as an important predictor of therapeutic response for chronic hepatitis C (CHC) patients receiving interferon-based treatment in 2009. Moreover, they also found that host genetic variations near IL28B gene also play an important role in the spontaneous clearance of HCV. On the other hand, inosine triphosphate pyrophosphatase (ITPA) gene variants are reported to affect ribavirin-induced anemia and therapeutic outcomes in CHC patients. In this article, recent advances in genome-wide association studies regarding HCV infection, and their impacts on current management of CHC patients will be reviewed. In addition, the clinical usefulness of genomic variations on the addition of direct antiviral agents (DAAs) to current standard of care will be discussed.

Keywords: Hepatitis C virus; Pegylated interferon; Viral kinetics; Metabolic profiles; IL28B SNP; Individualized therapy

ABBREVIATIONS

PEG-IFN: pegylated interferon;
RBV: ribavirin;
HCV: hepatitis C virus;
CHC: chronic hepatitis C;
RVR: rapid virologic response;
EVR: early virologic response;
ETVR: end of treatment virologic response;
SVR: sustained virologic response;
IL28B; interleukin-28B.

INTRODUCTION

According to the estimates of World Health Organization, approximately 180 million individuals worldwide are currently infected with hepatitis C virus (HCV). In addition, HCV may cause hepatitis, cirrhosis, as well as hepatocellular carcinoma (HCC), and is the leading cause of liver transplantation in Western countries [1, 2, 3]. Therefore, effective tackling HCV is an important health issue globally. However, previous standard of care for chronic hepatitis C (CHC) patients, pegylated interferon (Peg-IFN) plus ribavirin (RBV), is expensive, has many unpleasant adverse effects, and only effective in a certain proportion of CHC patients [4,5].

Table 1. Characteristics associated with virologic response in CHC patients

	Poor virologic response	Good virologic response
Host IL28B Genotype		
rs8099917		
G/T	G/G	T/T
rs12979860		
C/T	T/T	C/C
Other factors		
Viral kinetics	Non-EVR	RVR (+)
HCV genotype	1 or 4	2 or 3
Pretreatment viral loads (IU/mL)	>400,000	<400,000
HCV core protein	Mutant type (Gln70/His70)	Wild type (Arg70)
Ethnicity	African American	Asian
Liver fibrosis (METAVIR stage)	F3/F4	F0/F1
Gender	Male	Female
Age (years)	>40	<40
Metabolic factors	Obesity	
	Hepatic steatosis	
	Insulin resistance	
	Higher serum LDL	
Co-infection with HIV	Yes	No
Renal failure	Yes	No

For examples, the difficult-to-treat patients include HCV genotype 1 patients with a high viral load, HCV-infected African-American patients, and those who fail to achieve an SVR to previous interferon-based therapy [6]. Thus, identifying factors predictive of therapeutic response in CHC patients is clinically important in terms of increasing efficacy, avoiding unnecessary side effects, and saving medical expenditure. Currently, clinicians may use several predictors to access the benefits and risks of the therapeutic response in CHC patients, and advise patients who are likely to respond continuing treatment or stopping treatment in those who may fail. Of note, the number of these predictors is increasing, and several important predictors are identified in recent years. Consequently, personalized treatment for CHC patients is no longer a remote or impossible issue in the foreseeable future.

Several factors have been linked to the therapeutic response of CHC patients, including viral factors (HCV genotype, pretreatment serum HCV RNA titers, on-treatment viral kinetics [7], quasi-species [8], the polymorphisms in HCV core, ISDR or NS5A/B regions) [9-11], host factors [ethnicity [12,13], gender [14,15], metabolic factors [16,17], obesity [18], insulin resistance [19,20], advanced hepatic fibrosis or cirrhosis [21,22], steatosis [23,24], types of regimen [4], and duration of infection [25]. Among these factors, viral kinetics following antiviral therapy has been increasingly recognized as the most outweighing predictors of sustained virologic response (SVR) to interferon (IFN)-based therapy [26], and widely used in both clinical trials and daily practice [27]. For examples, the absence of an early virologic response (EVR) is the most robust means of identifying non-responders, and patients who fail to reduce serum HCV RNA by 2 logs or more at week 12 of treatment are likely to have non-response [28]. On the other hand, a rapid virological response (RVR), defined as undetectable HCV RNA at week 4 of treatment, using a sensitive test with a lower limit of detection of 50 IU/mL, can predict a high likelihood of achieving an SVR [29], and may be used as an earlier parameter in the hope of limiting exposure to and the side effects of therapy.

It is generally believed that host genetic background plays an important role in HCV infection, while the supporting evidence for this linkage is not strong. Although early genetic association studies have identified a variety of host genetic factors including single nucleotide polymorphisms (SNPs) of IFN response genes, human leukocyte antigens and T-cell immune response that may affect HCV infection or modulate the response of antiviral treatment [30-32], most of previous studies were limited by small sample size, indistinct phenotypes, statistical problems, or non-reproducible results [33]. Nevertheless, the situation changed in 2009. Several research groups simultaneously found a close link between the single nucleotide polymorphisms (SNPs) near IL28B gene (rs8099917 and rs12979860) and HCV infection in different HCV cohorts. These SNPs have strong impacts on treatment outcomes of pegylated interferon (Peg-IFN) plus ribavirin (RBV) therapy [34-38], HCV viral kinetics [39], and may partly explain the difference in response rates among African-Americans, Europeans and Asians

CHC patients. Moreover, these genetic polymorphisms are also significantly associated with spontaneous clearance of HCV infection [34]. On the other hand, different study groups also found inosine triphosphate pyrophosphatase (ITPA) gene variants may protect ribavirin-induced anemia [40] and affect the therapeutic outcomes of CHC patients [41]. All these lines of evidence not only provide us new strategies for the management of HCV infection, but also declare the beginning of genomic era in HCV studies.

In this article, we will discuss the impacts of these important host genetic variations on the management of CHC patients from three different aspects. First, we will review the recent advances of genome-wide association studies (GWAS) regarding HCV infection. Second, we will examine the usefulness of these genetic variations for the management of CHC patients. The last but not the least, we will foresee the clinical impacts of these genomic variations on the current triple therapy of direct antiviral agents (DAAs) in combination with Peg-IFN plus RBV therapy.

APPROACHES TO INVESTIGATE HOST GENETIC VARIATIONS

Host genetic background is known to play an important role in human diseases. The aims of genetic studies are to identify the susceptibility variants which may help us elucidate the novel mechanisms of disease pathogenesis, develop biomarkers for the evaluation of disease prognosis or treatment outcomes, and identify novel therapeutic targets [42]. Usually, we may use two different approaches to investigate the specific host genetic determinants: candidate gene or genome-wide approaches [43]. In candidate gene approach, the study is designed on the basis of a single (occasionally a cluster) candidate gene and the prior knowledge of disease process or gene expression. Genetic variants are identified through database searches or sequencing for the allele or genotype frequencies compared between cases and controls. Therefore, this approach is statistically effective, powerful, and may identify meaningful associations with the phenotypes of interest. However, as the selection of candidate gene is based on existing knowledge for the disease, it usually fails to deliver novel insights of the disease process

On the other hand, there are two different kinds of genome-wide approaches. One investigates the genetic linkage in families, and the other studies the genetic associations in populations of unrelated cases. In genome-wide linkage studies, the inheritance of chromosome regions which is more often than the expectancy in affected first-degree relatives is selected. Nevertheless, in genome-wide association studies (GWAS), the associations of large numbers of genetic variants and specific phenotypes in populations are examined without any prior hypothesis. Take advantage of the advances in genotyping technology and the availability of large databases for genetic variants, high-throughput genome-wide association studies (GWAS) may be performed easily than before and will become the main approach to examine the host genetic associations with diseases.

HOST GENETIC VARIATIONS AND HCV INFECTION WITH CANDIDATE GENE APPROACH

The Major Histocompatibility Complex (MHC) proteins may display fragmented pieces or antigens (self or non-self) on the host cell's surface to alert the immune system if foreign material is present inside a cell. There are two general classes of MHC molecules: Class I and Class II [44]. The human leukocyte antigen (HLA) molecules encoded by MHC class II which are found on macrophages, dendritic cells as well as B cells may present peptide epitopes to CD4+ T helper cells, and MHC Class I molecules may display intracellular viral proteins to cytotoxic T cells (CTLs; CD8 T cells) and natural killer (NK) cells. As both cell types are able to interact directly with infected hepatocytes, virus-infected hepatocyte is recognized and apoptosis through cell-mediated immunity [43,45,46]. For examples, many studies have identified the associations of HCV infection, T cells and MHC loci [47,48]. Activation of type 2-like T-helper (Th2-like) cells in acute hepatitis C patients is implied to play a role in the development of chronicity [49]. HLA-I-restricted, CD8+ T cell-mediated hepatocytotoxicity has been known as an important pathogenic mechanism in patients with chronic HCV infection[47], and the emergence of HCV variants with altered peptide ligands capable of antagonizing cytotoxic T lymphocytes (CTL) activity and a limited T-cell receptor (TCR) repertoire may provide a mechanism for HCV chronicity[50].

Since spontaneous clearance of viral infection is associated with vigorous polyclonal and multi-specific CD4+ T helper responses [51], several studies focused on this issue and found consistent associations of MHC alleles class II and HCV infection [52]. For examples, Tokushige K, et al found that TNF gene polymorphism and HLA-DRB1 haplotype may affect the activity of chronic HCV infection [53], and several studies have shown that MHC class II allele DQB1*0301 [48,54-56] and DRB1*1101 [48,52,57] are associated with the self-limiting HCV infection in different populations. Although one study in Taiwan has linked HLA class I and II alleles to the response to IFN-alpha treatment in CHC patients, and found that haplotype A11-DRB1*15 is associated with sustained response [58], studies for the associations of MHC alleles with treatment responsiveness and disease progression of HCV are largely inconsistent.

On the other hand, although viral infection is considered to be cleared by CD8-specific T cells by recognizing virus-derived peptide fragments presented with HLA class I, similar peptide-binding specificities of different HLA class I alleles, the diversity of study population, infection inoculums, and studies focused on single source outbreaks, have undermined the findings of strong associations in immunogenetic studies for HCV and HLA class I [43,46]. However, several studies have demonstrated the associations of resolution of HCV infection and HLA class I alleles. For examples, HLA-A*1101, HLA-B*57, and HLA-Cw*0102 are found to be associated with resolution of HCV infection [59-61].

As natural killer (NK) cells are a key component in the innate immune control of viral infections, and their functions are controlled by inhibitory receptors for MHC class I, including the killer cell immunoglobulin-like receptors (KIR) [62,63]. Several studies examined the associations of NK cells (and its receptors) and HCV infection. For examples, KIR2DL3 in combination with its cognate human leukocyte antigen (HLA)-C ligand has been linked to spontaneous resolution, treatment-induced resolution, and the so-called exposed uninfected individuals of HCV infection [64-66]. Moreover, cytokines also play important roles on the development of CD8- and NK-cell response. Polymorphisms within cytokine genes (such as TNF-α, TGF-β, IFN-γ, IL10, IL12, and IL18) have been associated with the spontaneous resolution, persistent infection, and treatment-induced resolution of HCV infection [32,67-71]. For examples, TGF-beta 1 functional polymorphisms, -509CC genotype and the -509C allele, are significantly associated with higher HCV clearance rates and with lower transcriptional activity [72], TNF-alpha promoter polymorphism at position -308 predicts therapeutic response of HCV-1 patients receiving combination therapy with high-dose IFN- alpha and ribavirin [67], and low CD83 expression as well as high IL-10 production of dendritic cells (DCs) at the baseline predict a poor virologic response to 24-week PEG-IFN plus ribavirin therapy in HCV genotype 1 patients [73]. Moreover, interleukin-1(IL-1)beta gene polymorphisms, IL-1beta-31 genotype

T/T or the IL-1beta-511/-31 haplotype C-T, are associated with hepatocellular carcinoma in patients with chronic HCV infection [74].

Of note, the functional significance of most the aforementioned alleles remains unknown [43], and the associations of alleles with HCV infection as identified by candidate approaches are not confirmed by subsequent GWAS studies.

GENOME-WIDE ASSOCIATION STUDIES IN HCV INFECTION

In 2009, several independent genome-wide association studies (GWAS) simultaneously identified the strong association between single nucleotide polymorphisms (SNPs) near interleukin-28B (*IL28B*) gene, encoding interferon-lambda-3 (IFN-lambda-3), and the response to interferon-based therapy among HCV-infected individuals [34-37]. In a total of 1,671 treatment-naïve Americans who were chronically infected with genotype 1 HCV and mostly were enrolled in the IDEAL study [75], Ge *et al.* [35] found a strong association of therapeutic response to PEG-IFN plus RBV with genetic polymorphisms near the IL28B gene. They also reported that the genetic polymorphisms near the IL28B gene are associated with an approximately 2-fold change in response to treatment, both among patients of European ancestry and African-Americans [35,36]. Among these polymorphisms, rs12979860 (located ~3 kb upstream of *IL28B*), which is in linkage disequilibrium with rs8099917 (located ~8 kb upstream of *IL28B*) (Figure 1), the SNPs identified by Suppiah *et al.* [36] and Tanaka *et al.* [37], respectively as the most strongly associated genetic variant with SVR. Among 191 participants of African ancestry in Ge's study, this association was about 3-fold (OR = 3.1, 95% CI 2.1–4.7), but the allele associated with treatment failure was more common in those of African compared to European ancestry [35]. In Tanaka's study, they enrolled 314 Japanese patients and reported a much stronger association with SVR (OR 12.1, 95% CI 6.5–22.4, compared to all non-responders) [37].

Although the results from this study may not be directly comparable to those from other reports because of the differences in study design, treatment agents as well as ethnicity, the magnitude of this odds ratio is remarkable, suggesting genetic variations near the *IL28B* gene may exert a stronger effect in Asian patients than those of European or African origin. In addition, Tanaka *et al.* [37] found a striking association of SNPs near the *IL28B* region to non-response (NR), which suggests that these variants may be associated most strongly with early response to interferon-alfa–based therapy. To clarify this issue, we enrolled 145 consecutive treatment-naïve Taiwanese CHC patients receiving Peg-IFN plus RBV treatment, and evaluated the impact of rs8099917 genotypes on these patients by using a new mathematical model [39]. We found that Asian patients with CHC receiving Peg-IFN plus RBV therapy have a lower daily viral production rate than Western patients, and the rs8099917 TT genotype may contribute to the better virological responses in CHC patients by increasing viral clearance rate.

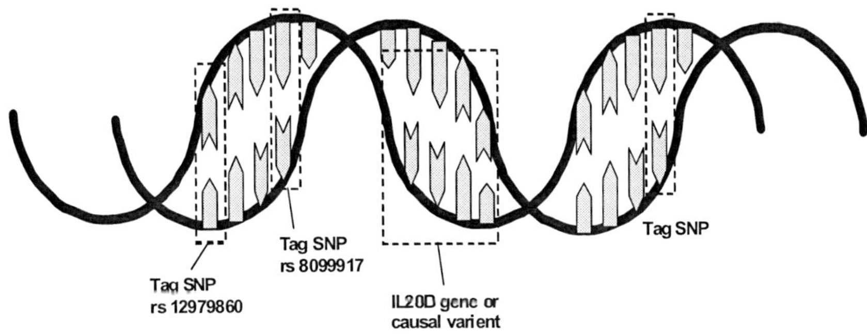

Figure 1. Tag single-nucleotide polymorphisms (SNPs) and linkage disequilibrium in a haplotype block.

In the meantime, Fellay et al. used a total of 1,602 DNA samples to study the genetic variants regarding RBV-induced hemolytic anemia, a clinically important condition. They found that genetic variants leading to inosine triphosphatase deficiency may protect against hemolytic anemia in hepatitis-C-infected patients receiving RBV [40]. Similar findings were reported from an independent cohort by Thompson et al. [76]. Ochi et al. also identified the missense substitution in inosine triphosphate pyrophosphatase gene (SNP rs1127354) may affect ribavirin-induced anemia in HCV-infected Japanese patients; however, they didn't identify ITPA variant rs1127354 had any significant association with SVR (P − 0.10) [41].

Although current GWAS studies provide overwhelming evidence that *IL28B* genotype is associated with treatment response to PEG-IFN/RBV for CHC patients, and differences in the frequency of unfavorable *IL28B* genotype may partially explain the different SVR rates among ethnicities [77]. However, the specific causal variants accounting for this effect and the pathophysiological mechanisms remain to be determined. Two studies found that the allele of rs8099917 associated with treatment failure was also associated with lower expression of *IL28A* and/or *IL28B* (both with similar sequences) in either whole blood [36] or peripheral blood mononuclear cells [37], suggesting a possible regulatory mechanism. Moreover, recent studies on serum IFN-lambda1 (IL-29) and IFN-lambda2/3 (IL-28A/B) levels in CHC patients with different outcomes demonstrated a higher IL-29 and IL-28A/B level in carriers of the rs12979860 C allele than in TT homozygous individuals (unfavorable *IL28B* genotype) (p<0.02) [78]. CHC patients had substantially lower serum IL-29 levels than healthy controls (p=0.005) and patients with spontaneously resolved hepatitis (p=0.001). In addition, patients with acute hepatitis C had intermediate serum IL-29 levels between those with CHC and normal controls; and patients who spontaneously resolved hepatitis C had higher serum IL-29 levels than those who became chronic.

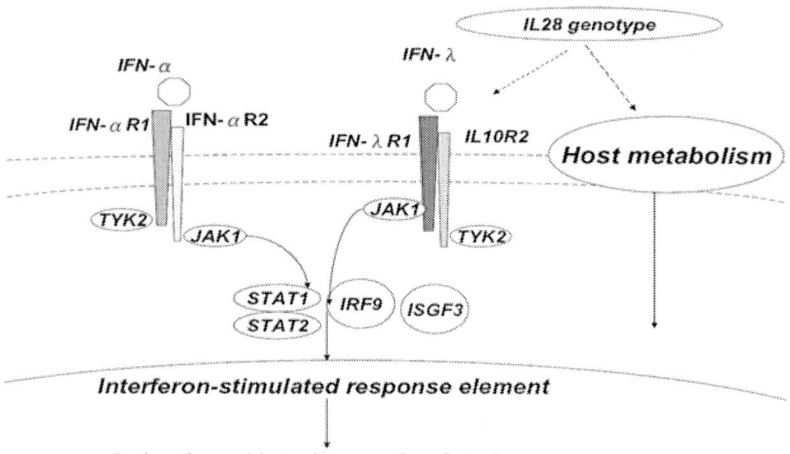

The interferon-ë proteins induce the JAK-STAT antiviral pathway by binding to different receptors than interferon-á, leads to upregulation of several hundred interferon-stimulated genes (ISGs), and some studies support this as a mechanism by which interferon-á and interferon-ë suppress viral infections and have demonstrated a link between IL28B genotype and ISGs in CHC patients. However, the link of IL28B and ISGs may be an epiphenomenon or at most only contribute a part of the link between IL28B genotypes and HCV, and an interaction on host metabolism may be a more proper pathophysiologic mechanism to explain the association between IL28B genotypes and HCV infection.

IFN, interferon; IRF, interferon-regulatory factor; ISGF, interferon-stimulated gene factor; JAK, Janus kinase; R, receptor; STAT, signal transducer and activator of transcription; TYK, tyrosine kinase.

Figure 2. Hypothetical pathophysiological mechanism of IL28B genotype.

They also found that HCV proteins NS3 and E2 may directly inhibit IL-29 production in poly I:C-stimulated purified dendritic cells (DCs). In addition, although some studies have shown that IL28B genotypes may partly explain the relationship of hepatic interferon-stimulated genes (ISGs) expression and treatment outcomes of CHC [79-81], our unpublished data demonstrated that metabolic factors may partly contribute to the incremental viral clearance rate of patients with rs8099917 TT genotype.

As there still no strong link was observed between IL28B and non-HCV subjects [82], and recent study also indicated that IL28B genotype was independent to hepatic expression of ISGs in CHC patients receiving IFN-based treatment [79]. Therefore, even some studies have demonstrated a link between IL28B genotype and ISGs in CHC patients [79-81], the link of IL28B and ISGs may be an epiphenomenon or at most only contribute a part of the link between IL28B genotypes and HCV, and an interaction on host metabolism may be a more proper pathophysiologic mechanism to explain the association between IL28B genotypes and HCV infection (Figure 2). Future studies are needed to clarify the pathophysiologic mechanisms of IL28B genotypes in patients with chronic HCV infection.

IMPACT OF GWAS FINDINGS ON INTERFERON-BASED THERAPY OF CHC

Although on-treatment viral kinetics (such as RVR or EVR) provides direct measurement of treatment response and is the most powerful predictor as well as key criteria for decision of continuing therapy, several important pretreatment clinical parameters (such as HCV genotype, viral load, age, sex, race, obesity, and insulin resistance) are also helpful to predict the treatment response and may be used to improve response-guided therapy (RGT) algorithms. Since host IL28B genotype is becoming the strongest host pretreatment predictor [83], the role of IL28B genotype in the decision algorithm regarding HCV treatment was examined. To clarify this issue, Thompson el al. examined 1,604 HCV genotype 1 infected persons from the IDEAL study [75] and found that CC genotype at rs12979860 was the strongest pretreatment predictor of SVR (odds ratio, 5.2; 95% confidence interval, 4.1– 6.7), and RVR remained the strongest predictor of SVR regardless of IL-28B type. However, the CC genotype was associated with a higher rate of SVR (Caucasians, 66% vs. 31% and 24%; P < .0001), implying that host IL28B genotyping may add further predictive power for patients who fail to meet current criteria used to predict therapeutic response.

In addition, several studies also examined the role of IL28B genotype in infection with different HCV genotypes, or HIV/HCV infection. Mangia el al. evaluated the effects of IL-28B polymorphisms on response to treatment with peginterferon and ribavirin in 268 genotype 2/3 patients (Caucasian: genotype 2, 213; genotype 3, 55) [84]. All patients were randomly assigned to receive standard duration (24 wk; n = 68) or variable durations of therapy. Patients who received variable durations (VD) and had a rapid virologic response (RVR) were treated for 12 weeks (VD12; n = 122); those without an RVR were treated for 24 weeks (VD24; n = 78). IL-28B genotypes (rs12979860) were analyzed for the association with treatment response. Although they found that differences between IL-28B genotypes were greatest among patients who failed to attain RVR (VD24 SVR rates: CC, 87%; CT, 67%; and TT, 29%; P = .0002), IL-28B genotype was not associated with SVR (>70% for all IL-28B genotypes) among patients with RVR (61%). In addition, Yu el al. examined the impact of several candidate SNPs on the treatment outcomes of 482 Taiwanese HCV genotype 2 patients treated with standard of care [85], and found that rs8099917 TT genotype is not associated with SVR, but is a significantly independent predictor for RVR, which is the single best predictor of SVR, in Taiwanese HCV genotype 2 patients. Taken together, these lines of evidence indicate that patients with HCV non-genotype 1 infection usually have a high rate of SVR, and IL-28B genotyping results may be more important for a subgroup of HCV genotype 2/3 patients without RVR.

Regarding HIV/HCV infection, Rauch el al. examined 1,362 individuals: 1,015 with CHC, 347 who spontaneously cleared the virus, 448 were co-infected with human immunodeficiency virus (HIV), and 465 receiving Peg-IFN/RBV treatment. They also identified rs8099917 G allele was associated with progression to chronic HCV infection (odds ratio [OR], 2.31; 95% confidence interval [CI], 1.74-3.06; P = 6.07 x 10(-9)). Moreover, they found the association in HCV mono-infected and HCV/HIV co-infected individuals were similar (OR: 2.49 vs. 2.16). Rallón et al. also examined the predictive role of rs12979860 SNP among 164 HIV/HCV-coinfected patients who had completed a course of Peg-IFN/RBV therapy [86]. They found that rs12979860 SNP was associated with HCV treatment response in HIV-infected patients with CHC due to genotypes 1 or 4, but not 3. These data highlight the importance of including IL28B genotyping as a part of treatment decision algorithm in difficult-to-treat population.

In conclusion, pretreatment clinical profiles including IL28B genotype, HCV genotype, viral load, age, gender, ethnicity, liver fibrosis stage, obesity, metabolic profiles and insulin resistance, may help on-treatment viral kinetics to predict therapeutic response and design the personalized therapeutic regimen. These clinical profiles not only provide a better assessment on the probability of therapeutic response and adverse effects for practicing clinicians, but also give us clues and chances to optimize the therapeutic response, especially for difficult-to-treat patients, who have a poor virologic response to current standard of care.

IMPACT OF GWAS FINDINGS ON NOVEL ANTI-HCV AGENTS

The introduction of direct acting antivirals (DAAs) will inevitably change the landscape of CHC treatment, especially in the USA and Europe where unfavorable IL28B genotypes are more prevalent. U.S. Food and Drug Administration (FDA) has licensed to two HCV protease inhibitors (boceprevir and telaprevir) for the treatment of CHC patients as part of a triple therapy with PEG-IFN/RBV in 2011. Promising results with improved therapeutic efficacy have been demonstrated in phase III clinical trials for treatment-naive and treatment-experienced patients with HCV genotype 1 infection [87-90]. However, increasing adverse events are concerned and have been reported in these studies [91]. Therefore, it is critical to select a subgroup of CHC patients who can benefit from the triple therapy.

Taken together, host genotype may provide additional important information to current response-guided decision algorithms for the treatment of CHC, and IL28B genotypes are shown to be useful in identifying a subgroup of non-RVR patients who are likely to achieve SVR to PEG-IFN plus RBV therapy. In the era of DAAs, host genotyping data could also play a role in optimizing the treatment regimen, duration, and the development of individualized HCV therapy (Figure 3). For examples, we can classify CHC patients into 3 different subgroups: easy-to-treat, intermediate-to-treat, and difficult-to-treat. When the treatment begins, on-treatment viral kinetic parameters are monitored and used to determine the therapeutic duration. If patients attain RVR or eRVR (extended RVR: i.e., undetectable serum HCV RNA level at week 4 and 12), a shorter therapeutic duration will be suggested.

                           Ching-Sheng Hsu and Jia-Horng Kao

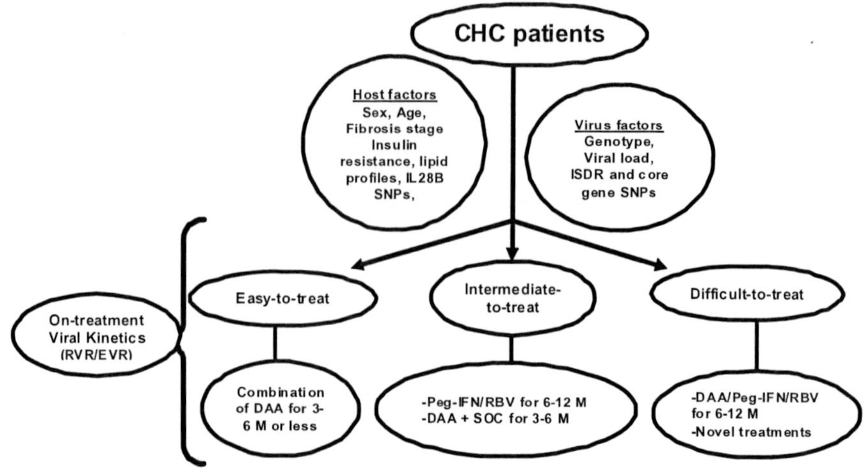

According to pretreatment host and viral factors, CHC patients may be classified into 3 different subgroups: easy-to-treat, intermediate–to-treat, and difficult-to-treat. When the treatment begins, on-treatment viral kinetic parameters are monitored and used to decide the therapeutic duration. If the patients attained RVR or eRVR, a short therapeutic duration will be suggested. In contrast, if the patients are non-RVR, but cEVR or pEVR, a longer therapeutic duration will be suggested. For examples, it is reasonable to suggest 3-6 months treatment for a person from intermediate–to-treat subgroup receiving triple therapy of DAA in combination with PEG-IFN plus RBV who attains RVR or eRVR. Although current guidelines suggest stopping treatment in patients who are non-EVR, whether it holds true in the era of host genotyping and DAAs remains unclear.

Figure 3. Hypothetical algorithm for personalized HCV therapy.

In contrast, if patients have non-RVR, but have cEVR or pEVR, a longer therapeutic duration or the addition of DAAs will be advised. Although current guidelines suggest stopping treatment in patients who are non-EVR, whether it holds true in the era of host genotyping and DAAs remains unclear. However, whether the predictive value of IL28B genotypes remains unchanged or might be weakened by the strong efficacy of DAAs awaits further studies. To explore this interesting and important issue, Akuta et al. examined the predictive role of IL28B genotype (rs8099917) in a Japanese cohort of HCV 1b-infected patients receiving 12-week or 24-week regimen of telaprevir/PEG-IFN/ribavirin triple therapy [92]. They found that the efficacy of triple therapy was high in the patients with genotype TT, who accomplished sustained virological response (84%), irrespective of substitution of core amino acid (aa) 70. In the patients having genotype non-TT, those of Arg70 gained a high sustained virological response (50%), and sustained virological response (12%) was the worst in patients who possessed both genotype non-TT and Gln70 (His70). However, more studies from different ethnic groups and DAA regimens are needed to validate their findings.

Recently, the strong link between genetic variations near the *IL28B* gene and CHC infection has attracted the interest in developing interferon-ë–based therapy for CHC patients [93]. An early clinical trial of pegylated-IL29 (interferon-ë1, or interleukin-29) reported antiviral effects among a small number of CHC patients [94]. An expected benefit is that the more restricted tissue distribution of interferon-ë receptors would result in fewer adverse effects compared to interferon-alfa. Although the preliminary results seemed promising, further large-scale clinical trials are required to confirm the clinical efficacy of pegylated interferon-ë for the treatment of CHC. Moreover, the usefulness of previously identified predictive factors for pegylated interferon-ë treatment remains unclear. Even though, current lines of evidence from GWAS results [35-37] and virological studies [95] all indicated the new treatment regimens including interferon-ë, pegylated interferon-ë or the combination of both interferon-alfa and interferon-ë, all of these regimens may be more effective and have fewer adverse events than PEG-IFN-based therapy.

CONCLUSIONS

Recent advances in the treatment of HCV infection have remarkably changed HCV infection to be a treatable and curable disease. Combining pretreatment clinical profiles and on-treatment viral kinetics together has substantially improved the accuracy in predicting therapeutic response and made personalized regimens become possible in the near future. As new DAA (such as boceprevir and telaprevir) become available, it may be prudent to defer current standard treatment and consider these new regimens for patients who are classified as "difficult to treatment" in areas where new DAAs are available. However, the availability of new anti-HCV drugs will gradually shrink the subgroup of "difficult-to-treat". Therefore, it seems to be the time considering the revision of our current recommendations for HCV treatment, which are based on the evidence regarding Peg-IFN/RBV and before the era of host genotyping and DAAs. Nevertheless, several important issues need be re-examined and revised thoroughly. For example, the treatment regimens, duration among different HCV genotypes and stopping rule for subjects without EVR. All these issues affecting our daily practice may be changed in the new era of host genotyping and DAAs. Finally, before the development of new consensus for the management of CHC, more studies are needed to provide solid evidence regarding the usefulness, benefits and disadvantages of these new therapeutic regimens as well as predictors.

DISCLOSURE OF CONFLICT OF INTEREST

All authors certify that all the affiliations with or financial involvement in, within the past 5 years and foreseeable future, any organization or entity with a financial interest in or financial conflict with the subject matter or materials discussed in the manuscript are completely disclosed (e.g. employment, consultancies, honoraria, stock ownership or options, expert testimony, grants or patents received or pending, royalties).

Ching-Shen Hsu: No financial interest related to the materials in the manuscript.

Jia-Horng Kao: Consultant for Abbott, Bristol-Myers Squibb, Gilead Sciences, GlaxoSmithKline, Merck Sharp and Dohme, Novartis, and Roche; on speaker's bureau for Abbott, Roche, Bayer, Bristol-Myers Squibb, GlaxoSmithKline, and Novartis.

ACKNOWLEDGMENTS

Grant/Funding Support: This work was supported by grants from the National Taiwan University Hospital, Buddhist Tzu Chi General Hospital, Taipei Branch, Liver Disease Prevention and Treatment Research Foundation, the Department of Heath, and the National Science Council, Executive Yuan, Taiwan.

All authors declare the independence of researchers from funders.

REFERENCES

[1]   Williams R. Global challenges in liver disease. *Hepatology*, 44(3), 521-526 (2006).

[2]   Kao JH, Chen DS. Transmission of hepatitis C virus in Asia: past and present perspectives. *J Gastroenterol Hepatol*, 15 Suppl, E91-96 (2000).

[3]   Chen DS. Hepatitis C virus in chronic liver disease and hepatocellular carcinoma in Taiwan. *Princess Takamatsu Symp*, 25, 27-32 (1995).

[4]   Strader DB, Wright T, Thomas DL, Seeff LB. Diagnosis, management, and treatment of hepatitis C. *Hepatology*, 39(4), 1147-1171 (2004).

[5]   Fried MW. Side effects of therapy of hepatitis C and their management. *Hepatology*, 36(5 Suppl 1), S237-244 (2002).

[6]   Ghany MG, Strader DB, Thomas DL, Seeff LB. Diagnosis, management, and treatment of hepatitis C: an update. *Hepatology*, 49(4), 1335-1374 (2009).

[7]   Hsu CS, Liu CH, Liu CJ *et al.* Factors affecting early viral load decline of Asian chronic hepatitis C patients receiving pegylated interferon plus ribavirin therapy. *Antivir. Ther*, 14(1), 45-54 (2009).

[8]   Fan X, Mao Q, Zhou D *et al.* High diversity of hepatitis C viral quasispecies is associated with early virological response in patients undergoing antiviral therapy. *Hepatology*, 50(6), 1765-1772 (2009).

[9]   Shire NJ, Horn PS, Rouster SD, Stanford S, Eyster ME, Sherman KE. HCV kinetics, quasispecies, and clearance in treated HCV-infected and HCV/HIV-1-coinfected patients with hemophilia. *Hepatology*, 44(5), 1146-1157 (2006).

[10]   Chayama K, Tsubota A, Kobayashi M *et al.* Pretreatment virus load and multiple amino acid substitutions in the interferon sensitivity-determining region predict the outcome of interferon treatment in patients with chronic genotype 1b hepatitis C virus infection. *Hepatology*, 25(3), 745-749 (1997).

[11]   Hsu SJ, Hsu CS, Liu CH *et al.* HCV core gene polymorphisms correlate with liver fibrosis but not sustained virological response in patients with genotype 1 infection. *Antivir. Ther*, 16(2), 227-235).

[12]   Lee SD, Yu ML, Cheng PN *et al.* Comparison of a 6 month course peginterferon alpha-2b plus ribavirin and interferon alpha-2b plus ribavirin in treating Chinese patients with chronic hepatitis C in Taiwan. *J. Viral Hepat.*, 12(3), 283-291 (2005).

[13]   Reddy KR, Hoofnagle JH, Tong MJ *et al.* Racial differences in responses to therapy with interferon in chronic hepatitis C. Consensus Interferon Study Group. *Hepatology*, 30(3), 787-793 (1999).

[14]   Berg T, Sarrazin C, Herrmann E *et al.* Prediction of treatment outcome in patients with chronic hepatitis C: significance of baseline parameters and viral dynamics during therapy. *Hepatology*, 37(3), 600-609 (2003).

[15] Backus LI, Boothroyd DB, Phillips BR, Mole LA. Predictors of response of US veterans to treatment for the hepatitis C virus. *Hepatology*, 46(1), 37-47 (2007).

[16] Hsu CS, Liu CH, Liu CJ *et al.* Association of lipid profiles with hepatitis C viral load in chronic hepatitis C patients with genotype 1 or 2 infection. *Am. J. Gastroenterol*, 104(3), 598-604 (2009).

[17] Ramcharran D, Wahed AS, Conjeevaram HS *et al.* Associations between serum lipids and hepatitis C antiviral treatment efficacy. *Hepatology*, 52(3), 854-863).

[18] Bressler BL, Guindi M, Tomlinson G, Heathcote J. High body mass index is an independent risk factor for nonresponse to antiviral treatment in chronic hepatitis C. *Hepatology*, 38(3), 639-644 (2003).

[19] Persico M, Capasso M, Persico E *et al.* Suppressor of cytokine signaling 3 (SOCS3) expression and hepatitis C virus-related chronic hepatitis: Insulin resistance and response to antiviral therapy. *Hepatology*, 46(4), 1009-1015 (2007).

[20] Hsu CS, Liu CJ, Liu CH *et al.* High hepatitis C viral load is associated with insulin resistance in patients with chronic hepatitis C. *Liver Int*, 28(2), 271-277 (2008).

[21] Heathcote EJ, Shiffman ML, Cooksley WG *et al.* Peginterferon alfa-2a in patients with chronic hepatitis C and cirrhosis. *N. Engl. J. Med.*, 343(23), 1673-1680 (2000).

[22] Myers RP, Patel K, Pianko S, Poynard T, McHutchison JG. The rate of fibrosis progression is an independent predictor of the response to antiviral therapy in chronic hepatitis C. *J. Viral Hepat.*, 10(1), 16-22 (2003).

[23] Akuta N, Suzuki F, Suzuki Y *et al.* Hepatocyte steatosis is an important predictor of response to interferon (IFN) monotherapy in Japanese patients infected with HCV genotype 2a: Virological features of IFN-resistant cases with hepatocyte steatosis. *J. Med. Virol.*, 75(4), 550-558 (2005).

[24] Patton HM, Patel K, Behling C *et al.* The impact of steatosis on disease progression and early and sustained treatment response in chronic hepatitis C patients. *J. Hepatol.*, 40(3), 484-490 (2004).

[25] Lin R, Liddle C, Byth K, Farrell GC. Virus and host factors are both important determinants of response to interferon treatment among patients with chronic hepatitis C. *J. Viral Hepat*, 3(2), 85-96 (1996).

[26] Fried MW, Hadziyannis SJ, Shiffman M, Messinger D, Zeuzem S. Rapid viral response is a more important predictor of sustained

virological response (SVR) than genotype in patients with chronic hepatitis c virus infection. *J. Hepatol*, 48 (Suppl. 2), 5A (2008).

[27] National Institutes of Health Consensus Development Conference Statement: Management of hepatitis C: 2002--June 10-12, 2002. *Hepatology*, 36(5 Suppl 1), S3-20 (2002).

[28] Fried MW, Shiffman ML, Reddy KR *et al*. Peginterferon alfa-2a plus ribavirin for chronic hepatitis C virus infection. *N Engl. J. Med.*, 347(13), 975-982 (2002).

[29] Jensen DM, Morgan TR, Marcellin P *et al*. Early identification of HCV genotype 1 patients responding to 24 weeks peginterferon alpha-2a (40 kd)/ribavirin therapy. *Hepatology*, 43(5), 954-960 (2006).

[30] Morgan TR, Lambrecht RW, Bonkovsky HL *et al*. DNA polymorphisms and response to treatment in patients with chronic hepatitis C: results from the HALT-C trial. *J. Hepatol.*, 49(4), 548-556 (2008).

[31] Welzel TM, Morgan TR, Bonkovsky HL *et al*. Variants in interferon-alpha pathway genes and response to pegylated interferon-Alpha2a plus ribavirin for treatment of chronic hepatitis C virus infection in the hepatitis C antiviral long-term treatment against cirrhosis trial. *Hepatology*, (2009).

[32] Yee LJ, Tang J, Gibson AW, Kimberly R, Van Leeuwen DJ, Kaslow RA. Interleukin 10 polymorphisms as predictors of sustained response in antiviral therapy for chronic hepatitis C infection. *Hepatology*, 33(3), 708-712 (2001).

[33] Clark PJ, Thompson AJ, McHutchison JG. IL28B genomic-based treatment paradigms for patients with chronic hepatitis C infection: the future of personalized HCV therapies. *Am. J. Gastroenterol*, 106(1), 38-45).

[34] Thomas DL, Thio CL, Martin MP *et al*. Genetic variation in IL28B and spontaneous clearance of hepatitis C virus. *Nature*, 461(7265), 798-801 (2009).

[35] Ge D, Fellay J, Thompson AJ *et al*. Genetic variation in IL28B predicts hepatitis C treatment-induced viral clearance. *Nature*, 461(7262), 399-401 (2009).

[36] Suppiah V, Moldovan M, Ahlenstiel G *et al*. IL28B is associated with response to chronic hepatitis C interferon-alpha and ribavirin therapy. *Nat. Genet*, 41(10), 1100-1104 (2009).

[37] Tanaka Y, Nishida N, Sugiyama M *et al*. Genome-wide association of IL28B with response to pegylated interferon-alpha and ribavirin therapy for chronic hepatitis C. *Nat. Genet*, 41(10), 1105-1109 (2009).

[38] O'Brien TR. Interferon-alfa, interferon-lambda and hepatitis C. *Nat. Genet*, 41(10), 1048-1050 (2009).

[39] Hsu CS, Hsu SJ, Chen HC *et al*. Association of IL28B gene variations with mathematical modeling of viral kinetics in chronic hepatitis C patients with IFN plus ribavirin therapy. *Proc. Natl. Acad. Sci. USA*, 108(9), 3719-3724).

[40] Fellay J, Thompson AJ, Ge D *et al*. ITPA gene variants protect against anaemia in patients treated for chronic hepatitis C. *Nature*, 464(7287), 405-408).

[41] Ochi H, Maekawa T, Abe H *et al*. ITPA polymorphism affects ribavirin-induced anemia and outcomes of therapy--a genome-wide study of Japanese HCV virus patients. *Gastroenterology*, 139(4), 1190-1197).

[42] McCarthy MI, Abecasis GR, Cardon LR *et al*. Genome-wide association studies for complex traits: consensus, uncertainty and challenges. *Nat Rev Genet*, 9(5), 356-369 (2008).

[43] Thursz M, Yee L, Khakoo S. Understanding the host genetics of chronic hepatitis B and C. *Semin Liver Dis.*, 31(2), 115-127).

[44] Complete sequence and gene map of a human major histocompatibility complex. The MHC sequencing consortium. *Nature*, 401(6756), 921-923 (1999).

[45] Bieber T. Atopic dermatitis. *N Engl. J. Med.*, 358(14), 1483-1494 (2008).

[46] Koziel MJ. Cellular immune responses against hepatitis C virus. *Clin. Infect Dis.*, 41 Suppl 1, S25-31 (2005).

[47] Liaw YF, Lee CS, Tsai SL *et al*. T-cell--mediated autologous hepatocytotoxicity in patients with chronic hepatitis C virus infection. *Hepatology*, 22(5), 1368-1373 (1995).

[48] Alric L, Fort M, Izopet J *et al*. Genes of the major histocompatibility complex class II influence the outcome of hepatitis C virus infection. *Gastroenterology*, 113(5), 1675-1681 (1997).

[49] Tsai SL, Liaw YF, Chen MH, Huang CY, Kuo GC. Detection of type 2-like T-helper cells in hepatitis C virus infection: implications for hepatitis C virus chronicity. *Hepatology*, 25(2), 449-458 (1997).

[50] Tsai SL, Chen YM, Chen MH *et al*. Hepatitis C virus variants circumventing cytotoxic T lymphocyte activity as a mechanism of chronicity. *Gastroenterology*, 115(4), 954-965 (1998).

[51] Ishii S, Koziel MJ. Immune responses during acute and chronic infection with hepatitis C virus. *Clin Immunol*, 128(2), 133-147 (2008).

[52] Thursz M, Yallop R, Goldin R, Trepo C, Thomas HC. Influence of MHC class II genotype on outcome of infection with hepatitis C virus. The HENCORE group. Hepatitis C European Network for Cooperative Research. *Lancet*, 354(9196), 2119-2124 (1999).

[53] Tokushige K, Tsuchiya N, Hasegawa K *et al.* Influence of TNF gene polymorphism and HLA-DRB1 haplotype in Japanese patients with chronic liver disease caused by HCV. *Am. J. Gastroenterol*, 98(1), 160-166 (2003).

[54] Cramp ME, Carucci P, Underhill J, Naoumov NV, Williams R, Donaldson PT. Association between HLA class II genotype and spontaneous clearance of hepatitis C viraemia. *J. Hepatol.*, 29(2), 207-213 (1998).

[55] Zavaglia C, Martinetti M, Silini E *et al.* Association between HLA class II alleles and protection from or susceptibility to chronic hepatitis C. *J. Hepatol*, 28(1), 1-7 (1998).

[56] Mangia A, Gentile R, Cascavilla I *et al.* HLA class II favors clearance of HCV infection and progression of the chronic liver damage. *J. Hepatol.*, 30(6), 984-989 (1999).

[57] Yenigun A, Durupinar B. Decreased frequency of the HLA-DRB1*11 allele in patients with chronic hepatitis C virus infection. *J. Virol*, 76(4), 1787-1789 (2002).

[58] Yu ML, Dai CY, Chen SC *et al.* Human leukocyte antigen class I and II alleles and response to interferon-alpha treatment, in Taiwanese patients with chronic hepatitis C virus infection. *J. Infect Dis.*, 188(1), 62-65 (2003).

[59] McKiernan SM, Hagan R, Curry M *et al.* Distinct MHC class I and II alleles are associated with hepatitis C viral clearance, originating from a single source. *Hepatology*, 40(1), 108-114 (2004).

[60] Thio CL, Gao X, Goedert JJ *et al.* HLA-Cw*04 and hepatitis C virus persistence. *J. Virol.*, 76(10), 4792-4797 (2002).

[61] Kim AY, Kuntzen T, Timm J *et al.* Spontaneous control of HCV is associated with expression of HLA-B 57 and preservation of targeted epitopes. *Gastroenterology*, 140(2), 686-696 e681).

[62] Orange JS, Fassett MS, Koopman LA, Boyson JE, Strominger JL. Viral evasion of natural killer cells. *Nat. Immunol.*, 3(11), 1006-1012 (2002).

[63] Cheent K, Khakoo SI. Natural killer cells and hepatitis C. action and reaction. *Gut*, 60(2), 268-278).

[64] Khakoo SI, Thio CL, Martin MP *et al.* HLA and NK cell inhibitory receptor genes in resolving hepatitis C virus infection. *Science*, 305(5685), 872-874 (2004).

[65] Knapp S, Warshow U, Hegazy D *et al.* Consistent beneficial effects of killer cell immunoglobulin-like receptor 2DL3 and group 1 human leukocyte antigen-C following exposure to hepatitis C virus. *Hepatology*, 51(4), 1168-1175).

[66] Romero V, Azocar J, Zuniga J *et al.* Interaction of NK inhibitory receptor genes with HLA-C and MHC class II alleles in Hepatitis C virus infection outcome. *Mol. Immunol*, 45(9), 2429-2436 (2008).

[67] Dai CY, Chuang WL, Chang WY *et al.* Tumor necrosis factor- alpha promoter polymorphism at position -308 predicts response to combination therapy in hepatitis C virus infection. *J. Infect Dis*, 193(1), 98-101 (2006).

[68] Huang Y, Yang H, Borg BB *et al.* A functional SNP of interferon-gamma gene is important for interferon-alpha-induced and spontaneous recovery from hepatitis C virus infection. *Proc. Natl. Acad. Sci. USA*, 104(3), 985-990 (2007).

[69] Mosbruger TL, Duggal P, Goedert JJ *et al.* Large-scale candidate gene analysis of spontaneous clearance of hepatitis C virus. *J. Infect Dis.*, 201(9), 1371-1380).

[70] Barrett S, Collins M, Kenny C, Ryan E, Keane CO, Crowe J. Polymorphisms in tumour necrosis factor-alpha, transforming growth factor-beta, interleukin-10, interleukin-6, interferon-gamma, and outcome of hepatitis C virus infection. *J. Med. Virol*, 71(2), 212-218 (2003).

[71] Yu ML, Dai CY, Chiu CC *et al.* Tumor necrosis factor alpha promoter polymorphisms at position -308 in Taiwanese chronic hepatitis C patients treated with interferon-alpha. *Antiviral. Res.*, 59(1), 35-40 (2003).

[72] Kimura T, Saito T, Yoshimura M *et al.* Association of transforming growth factor-beta 1 functional polymorphisms with natural clearance of hepatitis C virus. *J. Infect Dis.*, 193(10), 1371-1374 (2006).

[73] Liang CC, Liu CH, Lin YL, Liu CJ, Chiang BL, Kao JH. Functional impairment of dendritic cells in patients infected with hepatitis C virus genotype 1 who failed peginterferon plus ribavirin therapy. *J. Med. Virol.*, 83(7), 1212-1220).

[74] Wang Y, Kato N, Hoshida Y *et al.* Interleukin-1beta gene polymorphisms associated with hepatocellular carcinoma in hepatitis C virus infection. *Hepatology*, 37(1), 65-71 (2003).

[75] McHutchison JG, Lawitz EJ, Shiffman ML *et al.* Peginterferon alfa-2b or alfa-2a with ribavirin for treatment of hepatitis C infection. *N Engl. J. Med.*, 361(6), 580-593 (2009).

[76] Thompson AJ, Fellay J, Patel K *et al.* Variants in the ITPA gene protect against ribavirin-induced hemolytic anemia and decrease the need for ribavirin dose reduction. *Gastroenterology*, 139(4), 1181-1189).

[77] Conjeevaram HS, Fried MW, Jeffers LJ *et al.* Peginterferon and ribavirin treatment in African American and Caucasian American patients with hepatitis C genotype 1. *Gastroenterology*, 131(2), 470-477 (2006).

[78] Langhans B, Kupfer B, Braunschweiger I *et al.* Interferon-lambda serum levels in hepatitis C. *J. Hepatol.*, 54(5), 859-865).

[79] Dill MT, Duong FH, Vogt JE *et al.* Interferon-induced gene expression is a stronger predictor of treatment response than IL28B genotype in patients with hepatitis C. *Gastroenterology*, 140(3), 1021-1031).

[80] Urban TJ, Thompson AJ, Bradrick SS *et al.* IL28B genotype is associated with differential expression of intrahepatic interferon-stimulated genes in patients with chronic hepatitis C. *Hepatology*, 52(6), 1888-1896).

[81] Honda M, Sakai A, Yamashita T *et al.* Hepatic ISG expression is associated with genetic variation in interleukin 28B and the outcome of IFN therapy for chronic hepatitis C. *Gastroenterology*, 139(2), 499-509).

[82] Tseng TC, Yu ML, Liu CJ *et al.* Effect of host and viral factors on hepatitis B e antigen-positive chronic hepatitis B patients receiving pegylated interferon-alpha-2a therapy. *Antivir. Ther*, 16(5), 629-637)

[83] Thompson AJ, Muir AJ, Sulkowski MS *et al.* Interleukin-28B polymorphism improves viral kinetics and is the strongest pretreatment predictor of sustained virologic response in genotype 1 hepatitis C virus. *Gastroenterology*, 139(1), 120-129 e118).

[84] Mangia A, Thompson AJ, Santoro R *et al.* An IL28B polymorphism determines treatment response of hepatitis C virus genotype 2 or 3 patients who do not achieve a rapid virologic response. *Gastroenterology*, 139(3), 821-827, 827 e821).

[85] Yu ML, Huang CF, Huang JF *et al.* Role of interleukin-28B polymorphisms in the treatment of hepatitis C virus genotype 2 infection in Asian patients. *Hepatology*, 53(1), 7-13).

[86] Rallon NI, Naggie S, Benito JM *et al.* Association of a single nucleotide polymorphism near the interleukin-28B gene with response to hepatitis C therapy in HIV/hepatitis C virus-coinfected patients. *AIDS*, 24(8), F23-29).

[87] Jacobson IM, McHutchison JG, Dusheiko G *et al.* Telaprevir for previously untreated chronic hepatitis C virus infection. *N Engl. J. Med.*, 364(25), 2405-2416).

[88] McHutchison JG, Manns MP, Muir AJ *et al.* Telaprevir for previously treated chronic HCV infection. *N. Engl. J. Med.*, 362(14), 1292-1303).

[89] Bacon BR, Gordon SC, Lawitz E *et al.* Boceprevir for previously treated chronic HCV genotype 1 infection. *N. Engl. J Med.*, 364(13), 1207-1217).

[90] Poordad F, McCone J, Jr., Bacon BR *et al.* Boceprevir for untreated chronic HCV genotype 1 infection. *N. Engl. J. Med.*, 364(13), 1195-1206).

[91] Hsu CS, Kao JH. Boceprevir for chronic HCV genotype 1 infection. *N. Engl. J. Med.*, 365(2), 176-177; author reply 177-178).

[92] Akuta N, Suzuki F, Hirakawa M *et al.* Amino acid substitution in hepatitis C virus core region and genetic variation near the interleukin 28B gene predict viral response to telaprevir with peginterferon and ribavirin. *Hepatology*, 52(2), 421-429).

[93] Kelly C, Klenerman P, Barnes E. Interferon lambdas: the next cytokine storm. *Gut*, 60(9), 1284-1293).

[94] Muir AJ, Shiffman ML, Zaman A *et al.* Phase 1b study of pegylated interferon lambda 1 with or without ribavirin in patients with chronic genotype 1 hepatitis C virus infection. *Hepatology*, 52(3), 822-832).

[95] Marcello T, Grakoui A, Barba-Spaeth G *et al.* Interferons alpha and lambda inhibit hepatitis C virus replication with distinct signal transduction and gene regulation kinetics. *Gastroenterology*, 131(6), 1887-1898 (2006).

In: Hepatitis C Virus
Editors: A. P. Gonzales et al.

ISBN 978-1-61942-674-0
© 2012 Nova Science Publishers, Inc.

Chapter II

Hepatic and Blood Dendritic Cell Subsets in Patients with Chronic Hepatitis C Virus Infection

Aoife Kelly[1], Elizabeth J. Ryan[2] and Cliona O'Farrelly[1]
[1]School of Biochemistry and Immunology,
Trinity College, Dublin, Ireland
[2]Centre for Colorectal Disease, School of Medicine and Medical Sciences,
University College Dublin and St. Vincent's University Hospital,
Dublin, Ireland

ABSTRACT

Dendritic cells (DCs) are key mediators of innate anti-viral immunity being important detectors of viral infection and potent producers of Type I interferons (IFNs), IFN-α and IFN-β, as well as Type III IFNs, the IFN-λs. Successful adaptive anti-viral immunity also relies on the antigen presenting capacity of DCs and their production of cytokines that influence T cell polarisation. Defective immunity in patients with chronic Hepatitis C virus (HCV) infection has been proposed to be due to DC dysfunction which may also explain the poor success in generating therapeutic or preventative vaccination strategies for HCV infection. However, the many studies which have examined DC frequency and function in HCV patients to date have yielded conflicting results and the topic remains controversial. This may be because there are heterogeneous

DC populations including myeloid and plasmacytoid lineages with various subsets of DCs having functional specialisations and different tissue localisation. In addition, little is known about the DC subtypes that predominate in human liver, the primary site of HCV replication, with the major studies being carried out in mice due to difficulty in obtaining human liver tissue and isolating DCs. Here we review the literature on DC subsets from HCV-infected blood and liver and make suggestions for future studies in this area that might lead to an improved understanding of HCV immunity and provide us with additional therapeutic targets.

HEPATITIS C VIRUS

Chronic HCV infection is a serious condition affecting over 180 million people worldwide. The virus infects the liver and while it is estimated that 20% of those infected clear the virus spontaneously, the virus persists in the majority of individuals leading to liver fibrosis, cirrhosis and hepatocellular carcinoma as well as extra-hepatic manifestations such as lymphoma and mixed cryoglobulinaemia [1]. The current standard therapy of peg-IFN-α and ribavirin is only effective in approximately 50% of HCV genotype 1-infected individuals [2]. As yet there is no available vaccine for HCV and although progress has been made and more effective therapies such as protease inhibitors [3] are becoming available, it is still unclear why some people clear the virus naturally and respond to treatment whereas others do not. This variation in disease outcome and treatment response throws a spotlight on the roles of various elements of the immune response in clearance of HCV infection.

The major factors leading to HCV clearance are effective detection of the virus, an adequate innate immune response and the generation of an effective $CD4^+$ T cell response and IFN-γ production [4]. The initiation of T cell responses is dictated largely by the DCs. DCs are important phagocytic cells found in small numbers in the circulation and also throughout tissues regularly exposed to infectious agents e.g. skin, lungs, liver and gastro-intestinal tract, and were first described by Ralph Steinman in work which has just received the 2011 Nobel Prize in Physiology or Medicine [5, 6]. DCs detect microbes through expressing pattern-recognition receptors including Toll-like receptors (TLRs), C-type lectin receptors (CLRs), nucleotide-binding oligomerization domain (NOD)-like receptors (NLRs) and retinoic acid-inducible gene-I (RIG-I)-like receptors (RLRs) which sense pathogens, causing activation and maturation of the DCs and secretion of cytokines such as IL-12p70 required for a Th1 response. DCs, although rare, are considered the most highly specialised or 'professional' APC, capable of providing T cells with all three signals required for their activation [7]. DCs are also motile and, when activated following antigen capture, can migrate to the lymph node where they interact with T cells to mount an adaptive immune response. DCs process and present pathogens in the context of Major Histocompatibility Complex II (MHC II) but can also process antigens and present to $CD8^+$ cytotoxic T cells via MHC class I [8]. Another major function of DCs in terms of viral infection is production of Type I IFNs which are known to mediate the anti-viral responses by inducing the expression of hundreds of interferon stimulated genes (ISGs), among them, specific anti-viral genes [9]. Therefore, the cellular source and regulation of IFN production is an important question. While IFN-α can be produced by any virally-infected cell, it is known that plasmacytoid DCs (pDCs) are the major IFN-producing cells in the body, capable of producing 1000 times more IFN-α than any other cell type [10]. Aside from use of exogenous IFN-α therapeutically, the importance of IFNs in the immune response to HCV is underlined by the fact that the virus has evolved to target host signalling proteins (reviewed in [11]), limiting the efficacy of the IFN response and accounting for some of the treatment failure.

DENDRITIC CELL SUBSETS

Human DCs have been defined traditionally as $HLA\text{-}DR^+$ cells that lack the hematopoietic cell lineage (lin) markers CD3, CD14, CD16, CD19 and CD56. DCs can be subdivided into myeloid DCs or mDCs ($CD11c^+$ $CD123^{low}$) and plasmacytoid DCs or pDCs ($CD11c^-$ $CD123^{high}$) [12], with pDCs being traditionally defined as specialist IFN-producers whereas mDCs are potent antigen-presenting cells. Four additional surface antigens specific to human DCs are used to further distinguish DC subsets, Blood Dendritic Cell Antigen (BDCA) -1, -2, -3 and -4 [13]. Myeloid DCs can be divided into two subsets based on expression of either BDCA-1 (CD1c) or BDCA-3 (CD141) whereas BDCA-2 (CD303) and BDCA-4 (CD304) are expressed by all pDCs. The non-classical $CD16^+$ human monocyte are sometimes considered a blood mDC [12]. Blood DCs do not have the typical DC characteristics as seen in tissue DCs as they lack maturation markers such as CD83 and they lack dendrites. Blood DCs appear to only mature into functional DCs after entering the tissue [14]. In the skin, a separate DC subtype exists referred to as Langerhans cells, expressing langerin and CD1a. In the murine DC system, five DC populations can be identified in the lymphoid tissues of uninfected mice, segregated based on expression of CD4 and CD8 [15]. As with the human system, the major distinction can also be made between myeloid and plasmacytoid DCs, with myeloid DCs being further grouped into $CD8\alpha^+$ and $CD8^-$, with CD8 present as $\alpha\alpha$ homodimer rather than the $\alpha\beta$ found on CD8 T cells.

Table 1. Human blood DC subset nomenclature

DC subset	DC marker(s)	Marker function
Plasmacytoid DCs (pDCs)	BDCA-2 (CD303/CLEC4C)	Strictly expressed on human pDCs. CD303 (BDCA-2) is a type II transmembrane C type lectin. pDCs can uptake ligand via CD303 (BDCA-2) and process and present ligand to T cells [16]
Myeloid DCs (mDCs)		
mDC1 subset	BDCA-1 (CD1c)	Expressed on a major subpopulation of human mDCs (~0.3% of white cells) [13]. CD1c is a member of the CD1 family of proteins that are structurally related to MHC Class I proteins and mediate the presentation of non-peptide antigens to T cells [17]
mDC2 subset	BDCA-3 (CD141/ Thrombomodulin)	Expressed at high levels on a minor subpopulation of human mDCs (mDC2) (~0.02% of white cells) [13]. CD141 (thrombomodulin) was described to mediate co-agglutination by interaction with thrombin and protein C [18].

Further subtypes of $CD8^-$ DCs are based on expression of CD4. Other markers used for segregating mouse DC subsets are CD11b and CD205 (DEC205). The spleen contains three of these subsets; $CD4^-CD8\alpha^+$ $CD4^+CD8^-$ and $CD4^-CD8^-$ whereas the lymph nodes contain two extra DC subsets; $CD4^-$

CD8$^-$CD11b$^+$ and in skin-adjacent lymph nodes a further DC subset exists expressing high levels of langerin [15].

Many DC studies use murine models because of the difficulty in obtaining sufficient human tissue to study human DCs. Mouse DCs are generally isolated from secondary lymphoid organs such as the spleen or lymph node because the blood volume in the mouse is limited whereas human DC research has instead focused on cells expanded from blood populations. Frustratingly, while murine DC subsets have been revealed to comprise complex subsets, they do not match the human system, raising a question mark over the relevance of such studies in terms of human disease. A breakthrough in reconciling the mouse DC system to human was accomplished in 2010 with a series of papers published in The Journal of Experimental Medicine describing the human equivalent of a long-known mouse subset CD8α^+ [19-22]. This mouse subset, it is now agreed, is the equivalent of a tiny population of human blood DCs, CD141$^+$ or BDCA-3$^+$. These cells have yet to be fully characterised in human tissues but has recently been shown to be the most abundant DC subset in the lung [23]. The recognition of CD141$^+$ DCs as the human equivalent of CD8α^+ DCs has raised hope that studies of mouse DCs may translate to humans [24].

DENDRITIC CELLS IN HCV-INFECTED BLOOD

In all, the generation of a sub-optimal T cell response and defective IFN signalling in HCV infection has been hypothesized to be related to DCs. It has been suggested that the virus may possibly target the DCs, disabling their key function of linking innate and adaptive immunity through pattern recognition, T cell activation and IFN secretion. Numerous studies have been carried out on DC phenotype and function in HCV peripheral blood often with conflicting results (reviewed in [25]). Decreased numbers of myeloid and plasmacytoid DCs in the peripheral blood of HCV-infected patients compared to healthy controls is a consistent finding. However, numbers return to healthy control levels upon clearance of the virus [26]. Decreased T-cell stimulatory capacity, increased IL-10 secretion and a deficiency in co-stimulatory molecules on DCs in chronic HCV-infected individuals have all been described [27-32] but not all investigators are in agreement with these findings, with some concluding that DCs from HCV-individuals are phenotypically and functionally comparable to healthy DCs [33-35]. However, these studies have often been carried out on small patient

cohorts infected with different viral genotypes for different lengths of time
with varying degrees of disease progression and the presence of co-morbidities
such as alcohol use or co-infection with HIV or hepatitis B virus. Therefore
the topic remains controversial and requires additional study and further
necessitates the need to define the role of the localised liver DCs in chronic
HCV infection.

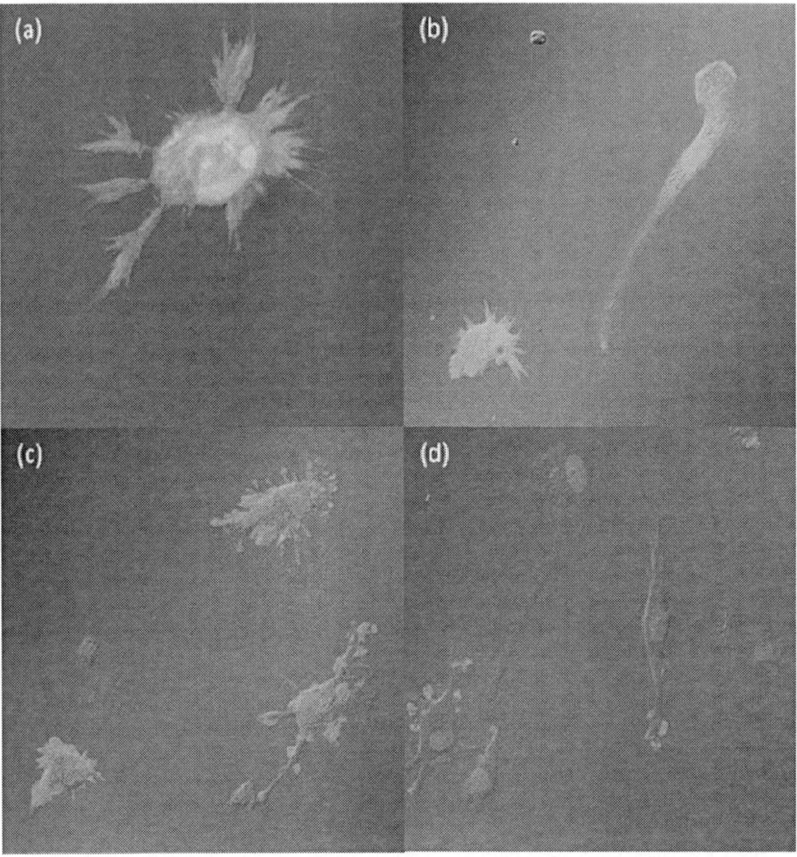

Figure 1. Myeloid-derived Dendritic cells (MDDCs) from Healthy and HCV Blood
Healthy MDDCs (a) stained with phalloidin (stains F-actin) show a contrasted
morphology to HCV DCs (b) which have a more elongated form. (c) Healthy DCs
express more DC-SIGN than HCV DCs (d).

Although blood is the most easily available human sample, it is becoming
apparent that although every organ in the body is 'bathed' in blood, each organ
has its own unique repertoire of DCs, influenced by the local

microenvironment, making it crucial to study cells directly from the organ of interest [36].

Progress has been made in this sense, with the advancement of techniques for the isolation of DCs and also the continued development of multicolour flow cytometry has also made more possible with DC immunophenotyping, with up to 12-colour protocols now available for DC characterisation [37]. However, detailed studies of DCs in HCV from the liver, the major site of HCV replication, are lacking.

DENDRITIC CELLS IN THE LIVER

The liver has its own unique immune system where cells differ from the periphery both in terms of frequency and functionality [38]. For example, large populations of innate lymphocytes are found in healthy liver including NK cells, NKT cells, iNKTs and $\gamma\delta$ T cells [39]. The immune system in the liver is required to tolerate many antigens translocated from the gut including dietary and commensal; it is therefore considered to be a mainly tolerogenic organ. On the other hand, this tolerogenic environment makes it an ideal hideout for many hepatotropic pathogens including HCV. However we do know that the liver is capable of generating successful immune responses as some individuals are capable of clearing the HCV virus naturally.

In relation to the supposed tolerogenic environment of the liver, an interesting observation is that liver transplants results in less rejection episodes than with other organs. Liver transplant recipients require a fraction of the immunosuppressive drugs, with reports of some patients being weaned off immunosuppression completely [40]. Furthermore, transplantation of another organ at the same time as a liver transplant makes it more likely that the other organ will be accepted, suggesting that the liver confers tolerance and may have a role in central tolerance in the immune system [41]. Among the prime candidates for the induction of hepatic tolerance are mDCs which govern the activation of T cell responses to being either pro-inflammatory or regulatory [42, 43].

To date, we have extremely limited knowledge about the frequency, phenotype and function of DCs in the livers of either healthy or HCV-infected individuals. Many hepatic DC studies have been carried out in mice, where it is agreed that murine liver DCs have an immature phenotype and therefore have tolerogenic properties, expressing lower co-stimulatory molecules, secreting lower IL-12 and being poor stimulators of naive allogeneic T cells partly because of low TLR4 expression leading to reduced capacity to activate T cells in response to LPS [44, 45] However, recent technological advances in DC isolation, increased availability of reagents for DC characterisation, along with the expansion of knowledge about human DC subsets [46] has given rise to increased interest in this area. Much of the difficulty in studying liver DCs is in the availability of sufficient liver sample from humans in order to isolate cells, especially given that DCs are present at such a low frequency. In particular, obtaining healthy human liver for research use is a difficult task as even the process of taking a liver biopsy is not without risks and complications [47]. In turn, while lymphocytes can be readily isolated from tissue, DCs are more 'delicate' and can be activated quite easily, changing their phenotype and making them difficult to analyse.

The limitations of studying human liver DC frequency and function are evident in studies such as that by Bamboat *et al* who utilised liver biopsies taken during liver resections from tumour-containing liver [48]. While care is taken to ensure that the biopsy is taken a good distance from the actual tumour, it is debatable as to whether this can actually be considered 'healthy' liver tissue as the presence of a cancerous tumour would induce changes in the whole organ. Different DC subsets were found in the liver and the blood, with BDCA-1^{+} mDCs being the most prevalent liver DC subset whereas blood consisted primarily of CD16^{+} DCs. Other subsets, BDCA-3 and the pDCs, had similar frequency in blood and liver. When stimulated with TLR4 ligands blood DCs produced pro-inflammatory cytokines but the liver DCs produced more IL-10 and as a result induced less proliferation of allogeneic T cells in a mixed lymphocyte reaction (MLR), instead promoting the induction of T regulatory cells (T regs). Increased IL-10 levels produced by liver DCs led to the generation of a substantially lower percentage of IFN-γ^{+} T cells thereby enhancing Th2 rather than Th1 polarisation. Liver DCs were also observed to be immature and inefficient at antigen capture and processing compared to blood DCs as measured by FITC-conjugating dextran and DQ OVA [48]. This recent human liver DC study was in agreement with an earlier report by Goddard *et al* who characterised liver DCs in comparison to skin using an overnight migration technique, whereby small pieces of tissue are cultured overnight, allowing cells to migrate out into the culture medium [36]. This method has the advantage of allowing the isolation of cells with minimal culture and cytokine treatments. This study also found that hepatic DCs produced higher IL-10 and were less effective at stimulating T cell proliferation compared to skin DCs, suggesting key differences between DC function at different sites in the body and further underlining the more regulatory or tolerogenic nature of hepatic DCs. Murine hepatic DCs have also been shown to be immature, capture less antigen and induce less T cell stimulation in comparison to splenic DCs [49].

Bosma *et al*, [50] utilised an alternative cell isolation method to characterise mDCs in liver by flow cytometry and immunohistochemistry. In this study, cells were isolated from *ex vivo* vascular perfusion of liver grafts pre-transplantation, a method previously exploited for the study of lymphocyte populations [51, 52]. The observation that the CD4/CD8 T cell ratio and the high percentage of NK cells in liver perfusate was the same as liver tissue strongly suggests that perfusate mononuclear cells are liver-derived, making it an ideal source to study liver cell populations including DCs [50]. Immunohistochemistry revealed the presence of BDCA-1$^+$ mDCs in the liver portal fields with few found in the parenchyma and functionally, these cells produced IL-10 and were of immature phenotype [50].

Most studies on DC frequency and function during HCV infection originates primarily from peripheral blood; paired blood-liver studies are required. While there is growing evidence that DC function is affected in liver disease, most work to date has been performed on non-hepatic DCs. DCs derived from blood precursors are unlikely to reflect DCs in the liver at the site of viral persistence isolated directly from the liver of HCV-infected individuals. It has been speculated that immune defects in HCV may be restricted to the liver and not reflected by changes in the peripheral department, thereby justifying the efforts to specifically evaluate liver DCs. Increasing knowledge of hepatic DC biology is likely to improve our understanding of HCV pathogenesis and therapy of liver disease [53].

Among the first studies to address hepatic DCs in HCV, Galle *et al* suggested a critical role for DCs in the pathogenesis of the immune infiltrate in chronic active HCV by demonstrating the presence of DCs as a regular component of the inflammatory infiltrate in chronic HCV liver in portal areas [54]. These DCs are present in contact with lymphocytes and hepatocytes and express T cell co-stimulatory and maturation molecules including CD83. Tanimoto *et al* similarly demonstrated the presence of mature activated CD83$^+$ DCs in areas of necrosis also containing T cells, with mild hepatitis having fewer CD83$^+$ cells than moderate hepatitis suggesting that an increase in DC recruitment or accumulation correlates with severity of disease [55]. In study by Wertheimer *et al* on DC subsets in blood, in addition to the study of peripheral DCs in a cohort of 112 patients, intrahepatic DCs were also studied in two patients, one of whom was chronically infected with HCV [56]. In the HCV patient, matched blood and liver studies revealed that mDC and pDC numbers were increased in the liver compared to the periphery. In another patient with non-HCV liver disease, there was an increase in mDCs but a decrease in pDCs. While this study was limited by low patient numbers, the results hint that there is specific accumulation of pDCs in the liver of HCV patients. An interesting finding was that patients with other type types of liver disease also had a depletion in their circulating DCs that was comparable to the HCV-infected group, suggesting that patients with any liver disease demonstrate diminished peripheral immune function.

Another HCV-liver DC study from the Adams group [57] utilised the 'walk-out' liver cell isolation technique allowing DC isolation without expansion by cytokines from human liver allowing study of un-manipulated tissue-resident DCs *ex vivo*. DCs from the liver of HCV patients were compared to non-infected, inflamed liver taken during diagnostic testing. Myeloid DC numbers in HCV liver were increased compared to non-HCV liver and demonstrated higher expression of MHC II, CD86 and CD123, were more efficient stimulators of allogeneic T cells and induced less secretion of IL-10. An IL-10 blocking experiment carried out on non-infected liver samples resulted in enhancement of the ability of mDCs to stimulate T cells, thereby suggesting that reduced IL-10 secretion in HCV liver may be a factor in the enhanced functional properties of mDCs from HCV liver. For functional studies, *in vitro* expanded myeloid derived DCs (MDDCs) instead of freshly-isolated blood DCs were used to compare to liver-derived mDCs which neglects to take into account the presence of more than one subset of mDC and is therefore a drawback of these experiments. It also was reported that pDCs were enriched in chronically inflamed livers compared to matched peripheral blood. Compared to non-HCV inflamed liver, pDCs were present at lower frequencies in HCV-infected liver. However, this group were unable to detect pDCs in donor liver which could be related to small sample size or the inability of the pDCs to survive in culture.

Nattermann *et al* [58] also demonstrated enrichment of DCs in the liver, with an elevation in the number of intrahepatic BDCA-1[+] cells, as shown using immunohistochemical techniques, in patients with chronic hepatitis B or C when compared with normal subjects. Here, it was also found that while HCV E2-induced RANTES attracts CCR5 immature DCs, the DCs are unresponsive to the CCL21 chemokine which prevents DC migration to the lymphoid tissue for interaction with T cells to generate an adaptive immune response. These data suggest that accumulation of DCs in the liver in HCV infection may be due to impaired migration induced by viral proteins, a concept also evident in a recent paper which showed that HCV E2 inhibited production of IL-2 and other cytokines by targeting the translocation of protein kinase C β (PKCβ), adding to the various mechanisms used by HCV to evade the human immune response and to establish persistent infection [59].

Table 2. Summary of Methods used to isolate Human Hepatic DCs

Method	Reference	Advantage(s)	Disadvantage(s)
Liver biopsy/ tumour resection	Bamboat *et al*, 2009 [48]	Accessible sample type	- Small sample size available - Presence of tumour effects overall health of liver organ
Perfusate	Bosma *et al*, 2006 [50]	Access to high cell number, relatively un-manipulated	- Not known if all representative DC populations removed from liver during organ perfusion
Cell migration	Goddard *et al*, 2004 [36] Lai *et al*, 2007 [57]	Increased cell number and less cell manipulation	- Possible that not all cell types migrate out - Some types of DC may not survive overnight culture
Immuno-histochemistry	Galle *et al*, 2001 [54] Tanimoto *et al*, 2001 [55]	Easily accessed material, retrospective studies possible	- Optimisation required - Unable to examine cell function

FUTURE DIRECTION

A recent breakthrough in reconciling the mouse DC system to human has led to renewed interest in DC subsets and their role in the immune response to infection and their therapeutic potential. The newly identified human equivalent of mouse CD8α⁺, the CD141⁺ DC subset, has yet to be characterised in human tissues. Astonishingly, this DC subset has been described to have quite a unique set of functions compared to other DC populations. Similar to the CD8α^+ DCs, human CD141$^+$ DCs have proven to be specialised in cross-presentation, making them an important cell type in the context of anti-viral and anti-tumour immunity [60]. While pDCs are specialised IFN-α producers and are considered at the forefront of DC anti-viral immunity, mouse CD8α^+ and human CD141$^+$ DCs appear to be the major producers of IFN-λ [61].

The novel IFN-λ family, consisting of IL-28A, IL-28B and IL-29, are suggested to have an important function in HCV due to the existence of single nucleotide polymorphisms (SNPs) in this gene region which have been shown in genome-wide association studies to be highly significant in determining the outcome to HCV infection [62-65]. This is the clearest genetic association with HCV pathogenesis to date but as yet the mechanism is unknown. IFN-λ is related to the Type I IFNs and IL-10, has been shown to be anti-viral and inhibit HCV [66, 67].

In contrast to the Type I IFN receptors which are expressed on most cell types, expression of the IFN-λ receptor, composed of the specific IL-28Rα chain and IL-10Rβ, is restricted to only a few cell types, primarily epithelial cells and pDCs [68, 69]. IFN-λ is being studied as an alternative therapy to IFN-α for HCV treatment as restricted receptor expression would predict fewer side effects [70].

Recent studies on IFN-λ see it emerging as possibly the most abundant IFN produced during HCV infection [71] but as yet a lot remains to be discovered about its biology. The identification of a novel immune cell type specialised in the production of IFN-λ is an exciting development in the study of its role in the immune response [61].

It has been suggested that IFN-λ produced by CD8α^+/CD141$^+$ DCs in secondary lymphoid organs may modulate innate and adaptive immune responses by acting either on pDCs or on other unidentified cell types [72]. In the study by Lauterbach $et\ al$ it was observed that the use of different cytokines, such as IFN-γ, and TLR ligands increase the production of IFN-λ in $vitro$ suggesting some form of interaction with other immune cells during poly(I:C) stimulation [61]. CD141$^+$ DCs and IFN-λ have therefore emerged as an novel immunotherapy target [72] and represent an exciting area of research. The development of knowledge about the different roles of DC subsets in the immune response could pave the way for therapeutic approaches based on direct targeting of specific DC subsets.

CONCLUSION

It is long accepted that DCs have an important role to play in anti-viral immunity, both in the generation of an adaptive immune response and in terms of IFN production. However, there is still little consensus as to the possible defects in DCs in HCV. Much of the study on this topic has been carried out on peripheral blood, in particular with exogenously-expanded MDDCs when in actual fact the primary site of HCV persistence is an organ with unique immunological make-up and properties that still remains to be comprehensively explored, in particular in terms of HCV infection. The discovery of new DC subsets in humans recently opens up to more possibilities of unknown cell types present in tissues such as the liver that have yet to be characterised, among them the elusive NK-DC cell type which has thus far only been described in the mouse [73, 74]. The expansion of knowledge about human DC subsets in recent years could mean that it may become possible to target specific DC subsets to generate an anti-viral immune response in the development of immunotherapy for the clearance of HCV and other viruses.

BIBLIOGRAPHY

[1]   Galossi A, Guarisco R, Bellis L, Puoti C. Extrahepatic manifestations of chronic HCV infection. Journal of gastrointestinal and liver diseases : *JGLD* 2007; 16(1):65-73.

[2]   Rosen HR. Clinical practice. Chronic hepatitis C infection. *The New England journal of medicine* 2011; 364(25):2429-38.

[3]   Ciesek S, Manns MP. Hepatitis in 2010: the dawn of a new era in HCV therapy. *Nature reviews Gastroenterology and hepatology* 2011; 8(2):69-71.

[4]   Thimme R, Oldach D, Chang KM, Steiger C, Ray SC, Chisari FV. Determinants of viral clearance and persistence during acute hepatitis C virus infection. *The Journal of experimental medicine 2001*, 194(10):1395-406.

[5]   Steinman RM, Cohn ZA. Identification of a novel cell type in peripheral lymphoid organs of mice. I. Morphology, quantitation, tissue distribution. *The Journal of experimental medicine 1973*; 137(5): 1142-62.

[6]   Steinman RM, Banchereau J. Taking dendritic cells into medicine. *Nature 2007*; 449(7161):419-26.

[7]   Reis e Sousa C. Dendritic cells in a mature age. *Nat. Rev. Immunol* 2006; 6(6):476-83.

[8]   Steinman RM, Hemmi H. Dendritic cells: translating innate to adaptive immunity. *Current topics in microbiology and immunology* 2006; 311:17-58.

[9]   Der SD, Zhou A, Williams BR, Silverman RH. Identification of genes differentially regulated by interferon alpha, beta, or gamma using oligonucleotide arrays. *Proceedings of the National Academy of Sciences of the United States of America 1998*; 95(26):15623-8.

[10]   Siegal FP, Kadowaki N, Shodell M, Fitzgerald-Bocarsly PA, Shah K, Ho S, Antonenko S, Liu YJ. The nature of the principal type 1 interferon-producing cells in human blood. *Science* 1999; 284(5421):1835-7.

[11]   Lemon SM. Induction and evasion of innate antiviral responses by hepatitis C virus. *The Journal of biological chemistry 2010;* 285(30):22741-7.

[12]   MacDonald KP, Munster DJ, Clark GJ, Dzionek A, Schmitz J, Hart DN. Characterization of human blood dendritic cell subsets. *Blood* 2002; 100(13):4512-20.

[13]   Dzionek A, Fuchs A, Schmidt P, Cremer S, Zysk M, Miltenyi S, Buck DW, Schmitz J. BDCA-2, BDCA-3, and BDCA-4: three markers for distinct subsets of dendritic cells in human peripheral blood. *J. Immunol.* 2000; 165(11):6037-46.

[14]   Ziegler-Heitbrock L, Ancuta P, Crowe S*, et al.* Nomenclature of monocytes and dendritic cells in blood. *Blood* 2010; 116(16): e74-80.

[15]   Shortman K, Liu YJ. Mouse and human dendritic cell subtypes. *Nat. Rev. Immunol.* 2002; 2(3):151-61.

[16]   Dzionek A, Sohma Y, Nagafune J*, et al.* BDCA-2, a novel plasmacytoid dendritic cell-specific type II C-type lectin, mediates antigen capture and is a potent inhibitor of interferon alpha/beta induction. *The Journal of experimental medicine 2001*; 194(12):1823-34.

[17]   Brigl M, Brenner MB. CD1: antigen presentation and T cell function. *Annu. Rev. Immunol* 2004; 22:817-90.

[18]   Conway EM. Thrombomodulin and its role in inflammation. *Semin. Immunopathol.* 2011.

[19] Bachem A, Guttler S, Hartung E, *et al.* Superior antigen cross-presentation and XCR1 expression define human CD11c+CD141+ cells as homologues of mouse CD8+ dendritic cells. *The Journal of experimental medicine 2010*; 207(6):1273-81.

[20] Crozat K, Guiton R, Contreras V, *et al.* The XC chemokine receptor 1 is a conserved selective marker of mammalian cells homologous to mouse CD8alpha+ dendritic cells. *The Journal of experimental medicine* 2010; 207(6):1283-92.

[21] Jongbloed SL, Kassianos AJ, McDonald KJ, *et al.* Human CD141+ (BDCA-3)+ dendritic cells (DCs) represent a unique myeloid DC subset that cross-presents necrotic cell antigens. *The Journal of experimental medicine* 2010; 207(6):1247-60.

[22] Poulin LF, Salio M, Griessinger E, *et al.* Characterization of human DNGR-1+ BDCA3+ leukocytes as putative equivalents of mouse CD8alpha+ dendritic cells. *The Journal of experimental medicine 2010;* 207(6):1261-71.

[23] Johnson TR, Johnson CN, Corbett KS, Edwards GC, Graham BS. Primary human mDC1, mDC2, and pDC dendritic cells are differentially infected and activated by respiratory syncytial virus. *PloS one 2011*; 6(1):e16458.

[24] Villadangos JA, Shortman K. Found in translation: the human equivalent of mouse CD8+ dendritic cells. *The Journal of experimental medicine* 2010; 207(6):1131-4.

[25] Ryan EJ, O'Farrelly C. The affect of chronic hepatitis C infection on dendritic cell function: a summary of the experimental evidence. *Journal of viral hepatitis 2011*; 18(9):601-7.

[26] Dolganiuc A, Szabo G. Dendritic cells in hepatitis C infection: can they (help) win the battle? *J. Gastroenterol* 2011; 46(4):432-47.

[27] Kakumu S, Ito S, Ishikawa T, Mita Y, Tagaya T, Fukuzawa Y, Yoshioka K. Decreased function of peripheral blood dendritic cells in patients with hepatocellular carcinoma with hepatitis B and C virus infection. *Journal of gastroenterology and hepatology* 2000; 15(4):431-6.

[28] Auffermann-Gretzinger S, Keeffe EB, Levy S. Impaired dendritic cell maturation in patients with chronic, but not resolved, hepatitis C virus infection. *Blood* 2001; 97(10):3171-6.

[29] Kanto T, Inoue M, Miyatake H, *et al.* Reduced numbers and impaired ability of myeloid and plasmacytoid dendritic cells to polarize T helper cells in chronic hepatitis C virus infection. *The Journal of infectious diseases 2004*; 190(11):1919-26.

[30] Tsubouchi E, Akbar SM, Horiike N, Onji M. Infection and dysfunction of circulating blood dendritic cells and their subsets in chronic hepatitis C virus infection. *J. Gastroenterol* 2004; 39(8):754-62.

[31] Ulsenheimer A, Gerlach JT, Jung MC, *et al.* Plasmacytoid dendritic cells in acute and chronic hepatitis C virus infection. *Hepatology* 2005; 41(3):643-51.

[32] Della Bella S, Crosignani A, Riva A, Presicce P, Benetti A, Longhi R, Podda M, Villa ML. Decrease and dysfunction of dendritic cells correlate with impaired hepatitis C virus-specific CD4+ T-cell proliferation in patients with hepatitis C virus infection. *Immunology* 2007; 121(2):283-92.

[33] Larsson M, Babcock E, Grakoui A, Shoukry N, Lauer G, Rice C, Walker C, Bhardwaj N. Lack of phenotypic and functional impairment in dendritic cells from chimpanzees chronically infected with hepatitis C virus. *Journal of virology* 2004; 78(12):6151-61.

[34] Piccioli D, Tavarini S, Nuti S, *et al.* Comparable functions of plasmacytoid and monocyte-derived dendritic cells in chronic hepatitis C patients and healthy donors. *J. Hepatol.* 2005; 42(1):61-7.

[35] Longman RS, Talal AH, Jacobson IM, Rice CM, Albert ML. Normal functional capacity in circulating myeloid and plasmacytoid dendritic cells in patients with chronic hepatitis C. *The Journal of infectious diseases* 2005; 192(3):497-503.

[36] Goddard S, Youster J, Morgan E, Adams DH. Interleukin-10 secretion differentiates dendritic cells from human liver and skin. *Am. J. Pathol.* 2004; 164(2):511-9.

[37] Autissier P, Soulas C, Burdo TH, Williams KC. Evaluation of a 12-color flow cytometry panel to study lymphocyte, monocyte, and dendritic cell subsets in humans. *Cytometry Part A : the journal of the International Society for Analytical Cytology 2010*; 77(5):410-9.

[38] Norris S, Collins C, Doherty DG, *et al.* Resident human hepatic lymphocytes are phenotypically different from circulating lymphocytes. *J. Hepatol.* 1998; 28(1):84-90.

[39] Doherty DG, Norris S, Madrigal-Estebas L, McEntee G, Traynor O, Hegarty JE, O'Farrelly C. The human liver contains multiple populations of NK cells, T cells, and CD3+CD56+ natural T cells with distinct cytotoxic activities and Th1, Th2, and Th0 cytokine secretion patterns. *J. Immunol.* 1999; 163(4):2314-21.

[40] Mazariegos GV, Reyes J, Marino IR, *et al.* Weaning of immunosuppression in liver transplant recipients. *Transplantation* 1997; 63(2):243-9.

[41] Rasmussen A, Davies HF, Jamieson NV, Evans DB, Calne RY. Combined transplantation of liver and kidney from the same donor protects the kidney from rejection and improves kidney graft survival. *Transplantation* 1995; 59(6):919-21.

[42] Thomson AW, Lu L. Are dendritic cells the key to liver transplant tolerance? *Immunology today* 1999; 20(1):27-32.

[43] Doherty DG, O'Farrelly C. Dendritic cells: regulators of hepatic immunity or tolerance? *J. Hepatol.* 2001; 34(1):156-60.

[44] Thomson AW, Knolle PA. Antigen-presenting cell function in the tolerogenic liver environment. *Nat. Rev. Immunol* 2010; 10(11):753-66.

[45] De Creus A, Abe M, Lau AH, Hackstein H, Raimondi G, Thomson AW. Low TLR4 expression by liver dendritic cells correlates with reduced capacity to activate allogeneic T cells in response to endotoxin. *J. Immunol.* 2005; 174(4):2037-45.

[46] Ueno H, Palucka AK, Banchereau J. The expanding family of dendritic cell subsets. *Nature biotechnology* 2010; 28(8):813-5.

[47] Bravo AA, Sheth SG, Chopra S. Liver biopsy. *The New England journal of medicine 2001*; 344(7):495-500.

[48] Bamboat ZM, Stableford JA, Plitas G, *et al.* Human liver dendritic cells promote T cell hyporesponsiveness. *J. Immunol.* 2009; 182(4):1901-11.

[49] Pillarisetty VG, Shah AB, Miller G, Bleier JI, DeMatteo RP. Liver dendritic cells are less immunogenic than spleen dendritic cells because of differences in subtype composition. *J. Immunol.* 2004; 172(2): 1009-17.

[50] Bosma BM, Metselaar HJ, Mancham S, *et al.* Characterization of human liver dendritic cells in liver grafts and perfusates. *Liver Transpl* 2006; 12(3):384-93.

[51] Jonsson JR, Hogan PG, Balderson GA, Ooi LL, Lynch SV, Strong RW, Powell EE. Human liver transplant perfusate: an abundant source of donor liver-associated leukocytes *Hepatology* 1997; 26(5):1111-4.

[52] Tu Z, Bozorgzadeh A, Crispe IN, Orloff MS. The activation state of human intrahepatic lymphocytes. *Clin. Exp. Immunol.* 2007; 149(1): 186-93.

[53] Lau AH, Thomson AW. Dendritic cells and immune regulation in the liver. *Gut* 2003; 52(2):307-14.

[54] Galle MB, DeFranco RM, Kerjaschki D, Romanelli RG, Montalto P, Gentilini P, Pinzani M, Romagnoli P. Ordered array of dendritic cells and CD8+ lymphocytes in portal infiltrates in chronic hepatitis C. *Histopathology* 2001; 39(4):373-81.

[55] Tanimoto K, Akbar SM, Michitaka K, Horiike N, Onji M. Antigen-presenting cells at the liver tissue in patients with chronic viral liver diseases: CD83-positive mature dendritic cells at the vicinity of focal and confluent necrosis. *Hepatology research : the official journal of the Japan Society of Hepatology* 2001; 21(2):117-25.

[56] Wertheimer AM, Bakke A, Rosen HR. Direct enumeration and functional assessment of circulating dendritic cells in patients with liver disease. *Hepatology* 2004; 40(2):335-45.

[57] Lai WK, Curbishley SM, Goddard S, Alabraba E, Shaw J, Youster J, McKeating J, Adams DH. Hepatitis C is associated with perturbation of intrahepatic myeloid and plasmacytoid dendritic cell function. *J. Hepatol*, Vol. 47. England, 2007:338-47.

[58] Nattermann J, Zimmermann H, Iwan A, *et al.* Hepatitis C virus E2 and CD81 interaction may be associated with altered trafficking of dendritic cells in chronic hepatitis C. *Hepatology* 2006; 44(4):945-54.

[59] Petrovic D, Stamataki Z, Dempsey E, *et al.* Hepatitis C virus targets the T cell secretory machinery as a mechanism of immune evasion. *Hepatology* 2011; 53(6):1846-53.

[60] den Haan JM, Bevan MJ. Constitutive versus activation-dependent cross-presentation of immune complexes by CD8(+) and CD8(-) dendritic cells in vivo. *The Journal of experimental medicine* 2002; 196(6):817-27.

[61] Lauterbach H, Bathke B, Gilles S, *et al.* Mouse CD8alpha+ DCs and human BDCA3+ DCs are major producers of IFN-lambda in response to poly IC. *The Journal of experimental medicine* 2010; 207(12):2703-17.

[62] Thomas DL, Thio CL, Martin MP, *et al.* Genetic variation in IL28B and spontaneous clearance of hepatitis C virus. *Nature* 2009; 461(7265): 798-801.

[63] Ge D, Fellay J, Thompson AJ, *et al.* Genetic variation in IL28B predicts hepatitis C treatment-induced viral clearance. *Nature* 2009; 461(7262):399-401.

[64] Tanaka Y, Nishida N, Sugiyama M, *et al.* Genome-wide association of IL28B with response to pegylated interferon-alpha and ribavirin therapy for chronic hepatitis C. *Nature genetics* 2009; 41(10):1105-9.

[65] Suppiah V, Moldovan M, Ahlenstiel G, *et al.* IL28B is associated with response to chronic hepatitis C interferon-alpha and ribavirin therapy. *Nature genetics* 2009; 41(10):1100-4.

[66] Robek MD, Boyd BS, Chisari FV. Lambda interferon inhibits hepatitis B and C virus replication. *Journal of virology* 2005; 79(6):3851-4.

[67] Marcello T, Grakoui A, Barba-Spaeth G, Machlin ES, Kotenko SV, MacDonald MR, Rice CM. Interferons alpha and lambda inhibit hepatitis C virus replication with distinct signal transduction and gene regulation kinetics. *Gastroenterology* 2006; 131(6):1887-98.

[68] Sommereyns C, Paul S, Staeheli P, Michiels T. IFN-lambda (IFN-lambda) is expressed in a tissue-dependent fashion and primarily acts on epithelial cells in vivo. *PLoS pathogens* 2008; 4(3):e1000017.

[69] Megjugorac NJ, Gallagher GE, Gallagher G. Modulation of human plasmacytoid DC function by IFN-lambda1 (IL-29). *Journal of leukocyte biology* 2009; 86(6):1359-63.

[70] Muir AJ, Shiffman ML, Zaman A, *et al.* Phase 1b study of pegylated interferon lambda 1 with or without ribavirin in patients with chronic genotype 1 hepatitis C virus infection. *Hepatology* 2010; 52(3):822-32.

[71] Marukian S, Andrus L, Sheahan TP, Jones CT, Charles ED, Ploss A, Rice CM, Dustin LB. Hepatitis C virus induces interferon-lambda and interferon-stimulated genes in primary liver cultures. Hepatology 2011.

[72] Luci C, Anjuere F. IFN-lambdas and BDCA3+/CD8alpha+ dendritic cells: towards the design of novel vaccine adjuvants? *Expert review of vaccines* 2011; 10(2):159-61.

[73] Shortman K, Villadangos JA. Is it a DC, is it an NK? No, it's an IKDC. *Nature medicine* 2006; 12(2):167-8.

[74] Crispe IN. Liver antigen-presenting cells. *J. Hepatol.* 2011; 54(2): 357-65.

In: Hepatitis C Virus
Editors: A. P. Gonzales et al.

ISBN 978-1-61942-674-0
© 2012 Nova Science Publishers, Inc.

Chapter III

Bone Metabolism Disorders in Chronic Hepatitis C Virus Infection

Germán López-Larramona[*1] *and Alfredo J. Lucendo*[2]
Departments of Internal Medicine[1] and Gastroenterology[2]. Hospital
General de Tomelloso, Ciudad Real, Spain

ABSTRACT

Hepatic osteodystrophy (HO) is an important complication of
chronic liver disease with an estimated prevalence ranging between 10
and 50%. Osteopenia and ostcoporosis associated to liver disease result in
increased morbidity due to bone fractures, chronic pain and immobility.
Cholestasis liver diseases such as primary biliary cirrhosis are the
conditions causing HO more frequently, but other liver diseases like
haemochromatosis, alcoholic liver disease and chronic viral hepatitis are
also responsible of bone impairment.

Loss of bone mineral density (BMD) occurs in patients with chronic
hepatitis C virus (HCV) infection, being more frequent and severe in
HCV cirrhosis with a prevalence of 20%-53%. The aim of this chapter is

[*] Corresponding author. Germán López-Larramona, M.D. Department of Internal Medicine.
Hospital General de Tomelloso. Vereda de Socuéllamos, s/n. 13700 Tomelloso (Ciudad
Real), Spain. Telephone: 0034 926 525 097; Fax: 0034 926 525 870; e-mail:
germll2003@yahoo.es

to summarize some practical issues regarding this topic and to provide a review about the main pathophysiological and therapeutic aspects.

Althought little is known about pathogenesis of HO in chronic HCV infection, it seems to be multifactorial. Bone loss occurs as a result of increased bone turnover and/or remodelling imbalance, being the latter caused by a reduced formation, an increased resorption or a combination of both. Vitamin D metabolism is impaired in the presence of severe HCV disease, and deficiency of this vitamin may cause hyperparathyroidism, increased bone turnover and accelerated loss of BMD. Disregulation of RANKL/OPG system, activated by cytokines involved in the pathogenesis of chronic liver disease (IL-1, IL-6, TNFα), is a defined mechanism for HO in HCV infection. Genetic factors such as polymorphisms of vitamin D receptor gene, collagen type Iα1 gene and the insulin growth factor-1 (IGF-1) gene have also been investigated and proposed to play a role in the pathogenesis of bone disease.

General management of osteopenia and osteoporosis in chronic HCV infection includes a prompt evaluation and an early diagnosis of osteoporosis using dual-energy X-ray absorptiometry (DXA). Application of therapy must consider general measures (correction of reversible risk factors, calcium intake and supplementation) and specific treatment for osteoporosis. Bisphosphonates are antiresorptive drugs that can improve BMD in other chronic liver disease, but only limited data are available for osteoporosis in HCV infection. Likewise, little is known about the effect of antiviral agents against HCV on BMD and their potential benefit on bone impairment. Orthotopic liver transplantation is followed by a transient BMD loss in the early months, but in the long term post-transplant there is a positive effect and a recovery of bone density.

Osteopenia and osteoporosis are common complications in chronic HCV infection, affecting both cirrhotic and non-cirrhotic individuals. The underlying mechanisms are not thoroughly understood. Thus, physiopathological bases of HO secondary to HCV should be clearly established in order to define specific treatments aimed at preventing and altering its clinical evolution.

ABBREVIATIONS

HO: Hepatic osteodystrophy;

CLD: Chronic liver disease;

HCV: hepatitis C virus;

BMD: bone mineral density;

PBC: primary biliary cirrhosis; PSC: primary sclerosing cholangitis;

OLT: orthotopic liver transplantation

1. INTRODUCTION

Hepatic osteodystrophy (HO) is the term that generically defines the group of bone mineral metabolism disorders, mainly osteopenia and osteoporosis, associated to chronic liver disease (CLD).

Osteoporosis is characterized by low bone mineral density (BMD) and predisposes patients to increased risk of bone fracture with high morbidity and mortality. Individuals with CLD have been described as having an increased rate of osteopenia and osteoporosis with variable incidence and prevalence rates among different studies. HO is therefore a common complication throughout the progression of chronic hepatopathy and involves deterioration in quality of life which affects the patient's long-term prognosis. Consequently, a detailed bone mineral density and bone metabolism evaluation should be performed in all patients with chronic liver disease in order to prevent fractures and chronic pain.

However, limited data are available on the contribution of chronic hepatitis C virus (HCV) infection to the development of bone disease in this group of patients. The aim of this chapter is briefly providing a general review of hepatic osteodystrophy in chronic HCV infection, focusin on epidemiology, pathophysiology and current therapeutic options.

2. EPIDEMIOLOGY. CHRONIC LIVER DISEASE AND PREVALENCE OF HEPATIC OSTEODYSTROPHY. PREVALENCE OF HEPATIC OSTEODYSTROPHY IN CHRONIC HEPATITIS C

Osteopenia and osteoporosis have become increasingly recognised complications among patients with CLD. Its etiology is complex and multifactorial and most of the knowledge relating to these disorders comes from studies conducted on patients with chronic cholestatic disease [1, 2].

Over the past decades several researches have been developed in order to estimate the prevalence and main changes in BMD affecting patients with CLD. However, the authors used different methods to analyze mineral density and they even have different definitions of osteoporosis, using parameters as fracture threshold or z-score [3-5].

On the contrary, more recent studies consider uniform methods measuring BMD with dual energy X-ray absorptiometry and defining osteoporosis and osteopenia according to the World Health Organization criteria. Following WHO guidelines, osteoporosis is defined as a T-score below -2.5 S.D. of the young adult mean value and osteopenia is diagnosed when T-score is between -1 and -2.5 S.D [6].

A high prevalence of osteoporosis is associated with chronic cholestatic disease (primary biliary cirrhosis –PBC- and primary sclerosing cholangitis-PSC-). This is one of the most widely studied group of patients with chronic hepatopathy in terms of bone mineral metabolism disorders. Its prevalence among different groups is estimated to range from 13% to 60% [7].

Various studies have been conducted on BMD of patients with PBC. The predominant alteration in these patients is osteoporosis, being osteomalacia very rare. Reduction in bone density is related to the severity of cholestatic disease, although not all patients with PBC develop osteoporosis and the rate of bone mass loss varies from one individual to another [8, 9]. Other factors linked to osteoporosis in PBC are the time to progression of the disease and the degree of cholestasis, as a reflection of the stage of chronic hepatopathy. Postmenopause and malabsorption of calcium in the intestine have also been suggested as predisposing factors in these patients [10].

The prevalence of osteoporosis in cirrhotic patients is related to the severity of liver disease expressed by Child-Pugh index [11-13]. This prevalence ranges from 20% to 50%, and inter-individual variations are observed in relation to bone density. The fracture rate ranges from 5% to 20% [14].

Alcoholism is an independent risk factor regarding the development of osteoporosis and osteoporotic fractures and has been especially studied in male patients. BMD of the lumbar vertebrae in these individuals is lower than in healthy controls [15], and the risk of fractures is independent from existing cirrhosis or associated hypogonadism [16, 17]. However, high alcohol intake in women who do not have cirrhosis and hypogonadism does not seem to be linked to osteoporosis [18].

The exact prevalence of osteoporosis in patients with CLD, but without cirrhosis, cholestasis or hypogonadism is unknown. The approximate prevalence of osteoporosis measured at the lumbar vertebrae in this group of patients ranges from 16% to 50% [19] with a fracture rate ranging from 12% to 18% [20].

Different incidence rates of HO have been described in patients with HCV infection. A study performed on a population of 72 patients with cirrhosis of different etiologies and Child stages (10 individuals with HCV-related cirrhosis) found an incidence of 100% for low BMD in the subgroup of HCV [21]. On the other hand, Nanda et al found no discernable bone disease in a group of 20 postmenopausal women with chronic HCV infection when their BMD was compared with two groups of patients with resolved infection and healthy controls, respectively [22]. However, the HCV-infection group showed a non-significative increased frequency of bone fracture (30%). Another study performed by Raslan et al on 30 HCV-infected patients (14 cirrhotic) estimated that osteoporosis of the proximal femur and lumbar spine was present respectively in 42.9% and 21.4% of the cirrhotic individuals [23]. Moreover, a significantly reduced BMD was described by Schiefke et al in a mixed-group of non-cirrhotic patients with chronic hepatitis B (n=13) and C (n=30). Low BMD was found in 58% of the patients and the rate of osteoporosis was 18.6%. Mean T-score value was lower in patients with chronic hepatitis C as compared to those with hepatitis B [19].

Like the whole group of patients with CLD, HCV-infected individuals may harbor additional risk factors for developing osteoporosis, such as hypogonadism, vitamin D deficiency, alcohol consumption, chronic steroid treatment and a low body mass index [24]. Osteoporosis predisposes to suffering bone fracture and increases morbidity and mortality. Vertebral fractures range in population with CLD from 3% to 18% [25, 26]. Therefore, HO should be early evaluated in chronic HCV infection in order to minimize risk of fracture and to improve quality of life and clinical outcomes [27].

3. PATHOPHYSIOLOGY: PATHOGENIC MECHANISMS INVOLVED IN BONE MASS LOSS IN CHRONIC HEPATITIS C INFECTION

Major factors influencing bone metabolism are genetic, but there are also essential factors like exercise, muscle activity, adequate nutrition, calcium and vitamin-D intake and a normal hormonal environment. Bone mass increases from childhood, approximately reaching maximum levels in one's thirties. From one's forties onwards, it starts to decrease in both genders but with a faster loss in women following the menopause. Peak bone mass is determined by the factors mentioned above. The rate of osteoporosis increases in the elderly as the loss of bone mass is a phenomenon associated with ageing.

Bone mass loss in CLD occurs as a result of an increase in bone turnover and/or an imbalance in bone remodeling. The latter can be caused by decreased osteogenesis, increased bone resorption or by a combination of both. Certain studies have shown increased bone resorption in the context of chronic liver disease, even in patients without osteoporosis. Other researches have shown a decreased bone formation [11, 28].

The risk of osteoporotic fracture is determined not only by bone mineral density but also by trabecular architecture, bone geometry, bone turnover and risk factors which are not associated with the skeleton such as postural instability and the risk of falls. The main risk factors for developing osteoporosis and, therefore, bone fractures in patients with chronic liver disease include: low body mass index (<19 kg/m2), excessive alcohol consumption, prolonged steroid treatment (5 mg/day of prednisolone for over 3 months), sedentary lifestyle, hip fractures in the mother at a young age (<60 years), hypogonadism and early menopause (under 45) [24].

Several pathogenic factors have been involved in loss of BMD among patients with CLD but few specific data are available for osteopenia and osteoporosis in chronic HCV infection.

Calcium and Vitamin D Disorders

Vitamin D is produced by endogenous synthesis in the skin, aided by sunlight, from which cholecalciferol is synthesized (vitamin D3). Both cholecalciferol and ergocalciferol or vitamin D2 can also be obtained from food. Vitamin D undergoes 25-hydroxylation in the liver tissue, a process which is affected by advanced liver disease.

Vitamin D deficiency is associated with secondary hyperparathyroidism, an increase in bone turnover and accelerated loss of bone mass. Fasting intact-PTH levels have been described in 42% of patients with chronic hepatitis C without differences among cirrhotic and non-cirrhotic patients [29].

Various studies have shown low serum 25-hydroxyvitamin D levels in individuals affected by chronic liver disease, with major decreasing as cirrhosis develops [21, 30, 31]. The main factors triggering vitamin D deficiency in chronic hepatopathy are believed to be limited exposure to ultraviolet radiation and nutritional deficiency. Intestinal malabsorption, alterations in the enterohepatic circulation of vitamin D and decreased skin synthesis in individuals with jaundice also contribute to vitamin D deficiency. However, no significant correlation between osteopenia and decreased vitamin D levels has been demonstrated in patients with chronic cholestasis [32].

Insulin-like Growth Factor 1 Deficiency (IGF-1) Deficiency

IGF-1 is involved in osteoblast differentiation and proliferation. Low serum levels of IGF-1 were observed in a study with bile duct-ligated rats, suggesting that cholestasis deeply affects its activity [33]. Therefore, its deficiency observed in cirrhosis and cholestatic hepatopathies may cause osteoblast dysfunction and osteopenia. Lower levels of IGF-1 and insulin-like growth factor binding protein 3 (IGFBP-3) have been reported in patients with liver cirrhosis due to HCV [23].

Receptor Activator of Nuclear Factor Kappa B Ligand (RANKL) and Osteoprotegerin (OPG)

The RANKL/OPG system regulates bone metabolism by modulating osteoclast activity, to the extent that OPG is a factor which inhibits that activity while the RANKL ligand activates it. Various researches have shown that the OPG/RANKL ratio is high in patients with chronic liver disease compared to control subjects, which shows that there is ligand consumption that activates osteoclastic activity, and an excess OPG as a compensating mechanism which tries to prevent the loss of bone mass [34-36]. Other cytokines involved in the pathogenesis of chronic liver disease such as IL-1, IL-6 and TNF-alpha can activate this system [7]. Additionally, circulating mononuclear cells could have a higher capacity to differentiate into osteoclasts in patients with chronic liver disease and osteopenia [37].

Hypogonadism

Hypogonadism associated with chronic hepatopathy has been proposed as a factor which favors the loss of bone mineral density. Low levels of estradiol, LH and FSH have been observed in postmenopausal women with cirrhosis, with normal testosterone and SHBG [38]. However, in males with advanced liver disease, there is an increase in the level of estrogen due to peripheral aromatization, which does not seem to protect against bone mass loss in individuals with alcoholic liver disease [39]. Other studies have shown that hypogonadism is common in male patients with cirrhosis but it is not correlated with osteoporosis [12, 20]. Moreover, recent researches suggest a protective effect of estrogens cirrhotic patients with normal BMD [21].

Hyperbilirubinemia

In vitro studies on animal models show that the increase in unconjugated bilirubin impairs osteoblast function in a dose-dependent and reversible effect [40, 41]. The results of research on humans are inconsistent. For some authors, osteopenia progresses at the same rate as jaundice does in patients with primary biliary cirrhosis and primary sclerosing cholangitis [42], while this correlation is insignificant for others [43].

Genetic Factors

Certain genetic polymorphisms have been proposed to have a secondary role in the development of osteoporosis in chronic cholestatic liver disease. These include the vitamin D receptor gene, the collagen type 1 alpha 1 (COLIA 1) gene and insulin-like growth factor (IGF-1) polymorphisms [44, 45]. However, no data are available for genetic factors influencing osteoporosis development in chronic HCV infection.

Lifestyle Factors

Concomitant alcohol intake or tobacco consumption may aggravate HO in patients with chronic hepatitis C, together with a sedentary lifestyle, malnutrition and a low body mass index [46].

DIAGNOSIS OF HEPATIC OSTEODYSTROPHY IN CHRONIC HEPATITIS C

The main objective for assessing and treating hepatic osteodystrophy is to prevent bone fractures and, thus, to achieve a better quality of life for individuals with chronic liver disease.

As noted before, bone mineral density is measured using dual energy X-ray bone absorptiometry performed on the lumbar vertebrae and femoral neck. The results of the measurement are classified on a scale by the WHO, the *T-score* being the basic parameter for diagnosis. Osteoporosis is therefore defined as a BMD of less than 2.5 standard deviation compared to the normal average score for young adults (*T-score* of less than -2.5). Similarly, osteopenia is defined as having a *T-score* of between -1 and -2.5 [6]. Prospective studies in cholestatic liver disease show how the risk of fractures increases progressively in proportion to the decrease in BMD, with a two-fold to three-fold increase per standard deviation decrease therein [47].

In view of the close relationship between chronic hepatitis C infection and bone metabolism disorders, assessment of osteopenia and osteoporosis in this group of patients should be mandatory [48-50]. Consequently, hemogram and basic biochemistry tests including liver function, phosphocalcic metabolism, gonadal and thyroid hormones must be drawn. In addition to analytical parameters, bone absorptiometry must be performed on lumbar spine and femoral neck [24]. A simple X-ray of the dorsal and lumbar vertebrae is indicated if there is a clinical suspicion of spinal fracture, as this is an indication for treatment, irrespective of bone density [51].

Systematic determination of bone turnover markers (BTM) in order to assess bone impairment in chronic liver disease remains controversial. During the bone-remodeling process, enzymes and non-enzymatic peptides reach the bloodstream and/or are eliminated through urine. Their concentration in blood and urine is related to the total bone turnover rate. BTM can be divided in two groups: bone resorption markers (e.g. procollagen type 1 carboxyterminal and aminoterminal propeptides, osteocalcin and alkaline phosphatase bone isoenzyme) and bone formation markers (e.g. deoxypyridinoline, pyridinoline, type-1 collagen amino-terminal telopeptide). BTM levels are higher in patients with osteoporosis and there is an inverse relationship between their levels and BMD. Literature shows different studies including patients with chronic hepatitis C whose levels of BTM were determined. Some of them describe a BTM pattern of increased resorption [21] while others found high levels of formation BTM [19] or no significative differences between both subgroups of BTM [22]. Hence, there is neither particular consensus nor an appropriate recommendation based on clinical practice guidelines about their use in clinical management of patients with hepatitis C and HO. It is thought that BTM could be useful for monitoring bone mass loss in response to treatment for osteoporosis and for predicting fracture risk, but this potential application should be verified due to the fact that they have been researched only in few studies with patients suffering from chronic liver disease [52, 53]. Furthermore, BTM levels in CLD may be influenced by the extent of hepatic fibrosis and by intrahepatic metabolism of collagen, making it difficult to interpret the results obtained [24].

THERAPEUTIC MANAGEMENT OF HEPATIC OSTEODYSTROPHY IN CHRONIC HEPATITIS C

Little evidence is available about specific therapy of HO in chronic hepatitis C. Most of the researches have been performed on patients with chronic cholestatic liver disease. Besides, there is a lack of randomized-controlled intervention studies on the prevention of osteoporosis and bone fractures in CLD. Consequently, most of the general and specific treatments described below will be referred to those available for general HO.

General Measures. Vitamin D and Calcium Supplementation

Lifestyle and nutritional measures aimed at correcting reversible risk factors for osteoporosis must be always implemented. Patients will be encouraged to avoid smoking and alcohol consumption and to practice moderate physical activity.

Extensive studies have provided no evidence on the effect of calcium and vitamin D in preventing OP and fractures in these patients. Research has been performed on small groups yielding inconsistent BMD results [8, 30, 47]. However, it seems reasonable to recommend supplements by taking a daily dose of 800 UI of vitamin D3 and 1g of calcium [24, 51].

Anti-osteoporotic Drugs in the Treatment of Hepatic Osteodystrophy

Nowadays, bisphosphonates are the main pharmacological agents used in the treatment of hepatic osteodistrophy, despite the fact that limited data on bisphosphonates-therapy in chronic liver disease are available. Bisphosphonates selectively inhibit osteoclast activity with a potent anti-resorptive effect. These agents reduce the risk of vertebral and non-vertebral fractures and increase BMD in postmenopausal osteoporotic women without liver disease [39]. They also have shown to be effective in preventing steroid-induced osteoporosis in primary biliary cirrhosis [3]. However, there is a lack of long-term controlled studies developed to evaluate the efficiency of bisphosphonates in fracture-prevention in individuals with CLD. A study with 80 post-menopausal women with osteoporosis and chronic liver disease secondary to hepatitis virus B and C suggests that a cyclic etidronate treatment could be effective to reduce the incidence of bone fracture [54]. Alendronate is capable to improve BMD of patients with primary biliary cirrhosis [55, 56], although caution is required because of potential esophageal side effects [24]. Risedronate seems to have a less toxic effect on the esophageal mucosa, which could be useful for treating patients with esophageal varices. Hence, bisphosphonates are the choice agents that should be used in the setting of HO in chronic HCV infection, although limited evidence is available in this group of patients [24, 51].

Hormone replacement with testosterone in hypogonadic males without CLD was efficient and increased BMD in a study on 11 men with primary and secondary hypogonadism [57]. Nonetheless, treatment of hypogonadism in the setting of CLD and HO remains as a controversial decision. Hormonal replacement with estrogen and progesterone emerged as a safe treatment for women with CLD, administered either orally or transdermally and sequentially or continuously [58, 59]. Following the publication of the HERS II [60] and WHI [61] studies questioning the safety of this therapy, its use is currently not recommended . The increased risk of hepatocellular carcinoma related to this treatment should be also taken into account, by weighing up the relationship between its benefits and risks and it should be better administered transdermally [7, 24, 51].

Other antiosteoporotic drugs such as parathyroid hormone and raloxifene have been evaluated in chronic cholestatic disease [62] and in animal models [63], but there are no data from randomized studies about treatment of HO in chronic hepatitis C.

Antiviral Drugs and their Effect on BMD

Current combinated therapies against HCV based on interferon-alpha plus ribavirin have led to a significative improvement in sustained virological response rates [64].

However, harmful secondary effects on BMD due to antiviral agents have been described. Solís-Herruzo et al found a significantly lower BMD in 19 male patients treated for 12 months with interferon plus ribavirin, when compared with BMD in a matched interferon-monotherapy group [65]. *In vitro* studies suggest that ribavirin may induce a failure in osteoblasts differentiation in a time and dose-dependent way [66]. More recent researches have reported a ribavirin-induced osteoclasts formation through osteoblasts via up-regulation of TRANCE/RANKL gene expression [67]. On the other hand, some clinical studies have found no negative effects of ribavirin on bone density [68]. Furthermore, an on-treatment increasing of BMD has been reported by Hoffmann et al. in a study on 30 patients with genotype-1 chronic HCV infection treated with pegylated interferon alpha and ribavirin [69]. A retrospective study by Arase et al. on 420 postmenopausal women with chronic HCV infection treated with interferon-monotherapy reported that virus clearance caused a two-thirds reduction in the risk of bone fracture, with a cumulative 10-years risk of 9.2% [70].

Thus, further research is required in order to determine whether antiviral therapy may induce a significative bone loss in HCV-infected patients.

Orthotopic Liver Transplantation and Bone Mineral Density in Chronic Hepatitis C

Orthotopic liver transplantation (OLT) is the treatment of choice for end-stage liver disease secondáry to chronic HCV infection [64]. Patients awaiting liver transplantation have a high rate of BMD loss, with a significative prevalence of osteopenia and osteoporosis (26-33% and 11.5-42%, respectively) [71]. Significant decreases in BMD may occur in the first three to six months following OLT, with an increased estimated rate of bone fracture (17.2-42%) [72].

Nevertheless, there is a lack of specific trials evaluating BMD loss and its management in HCV patients after OLT. This is the reason why BMD disorders in transplant HCV-infected recipients should be managed according to data from available evidence.

The predominant pathogenic mechanism for bone loss after OLT seems to be an excess of bone resorption as shown in small studies including heterogeneous groups of patients with CLD who underwent OLT [73, 74]. In the same way, a low preoperative BMD may predispose to bone fracture postoperatively [75]. More than 3-6 months after OLT, BMD remains stable or gradually increases [74, 76]. An improvement in spinal density was reported by Eastell et al. in a study with BMD measurements after OLT in patients with chronic cholestatic disease [77]. In the same way, Guichelaar et al described an improvement in osteopenia rates after OLT in a prospective study of patients with primary biliary cirrhosis and primary sclerosing cholangitis [78].

Preventive strategies and specific antiresorptive therapy should be implemented in post-OLT patients, in order to minimize bone loss. Corticosteroid therapy in transplant recipients should be carefully adjusted to the minimum effective dosage [79]. Bisphosphonates are useful antiresorptive drugs capable of avoiding bone loss after OLT [79-81], without a clear evidence to consider a specific bisphosphonate as first line therapy. Other agents such as calcitonin have been tested in post-OLT patients, showing a less potent antiresorptive effect than bisphosphonates [82].

CONCLUSIONS

HO is a frequent disorder in patients with chronic liver disease secondary to HCV infection. Osteopenia and osteoporosis develop as a result of multiple pathogenic mechanisms and a disregulation of bone formation and resorption. A global approach in the setting of liver disease secondary to HCV is required in order to consider and prevent HO as a potential complication of the whole disease. Further investigation is needed to achieve a better understanding of physiopatological mechanisms. Moreover, evidence from randomized and multicentric studies should be desiderable to evaluate the best treatment alternatives capable of avoiding bone loss in the different stages of chronic HCV infection.

REFERENCES

[1] Rouillard S, Lane NE. Hepatic osteodystrophy. *Hepatology* 2001;33:301-307.

[2] Pusl T, Beuers U. Extrahepatic manifestations of cholestatic liver diseases, pathogenesis and therapy. *Clin Rev Allerg Immunol* 2005;28:147-157.

[3] Wolfhagen FH, van Buuren HR, den Ouden JW, Hop WC, van Leeuwen JP, Schalm SW, Pols HA. Cyclical etidronate in the prevention of bone loss in corticosteroid-treated primary biliary cirrhosis. A prospective, controlled pilot study. *J Hepatol* 1997;26:325-330.

[4] Matloff DS, Kaplan, M, Neer RM, Goldberg MJ, Bitman W, Wolfe HJ. Osteoporosis in primary biliary cirrhosis: effects of 25-hydroxyvitamin D3 treatment. *Gastroenterology* 1982;83:97-102.

[5] Epstein O, Kato Y, Dick R, Sherlock S. Vitamin D, hydroxyapatite, and calcium gluconate in treatment of cortical bone thinning in postmenopausal women with primary biliary cirrhosis. *Am J Clin Nutr* 1982;36:426-430.

[6] Report of WHO Study Group. Assessment of fracture risk and its application to screening for postmenopausal osteoporosis. World Health *Organ Tech Rep Ser* 1994;843:1-129.

[7] Gasser RW. Cholestasis and metabolic bone disease - a clinical review. *Wien Med Wochenschr* 2008;158:553-557.

[8] Van Berkum FN, Beukers R, Birkenhäger JC, Kooij PP, Schalm SW, Pols A. Bone mass in women with primary biliary cirrhosis: the relation with histological stage and the use of steroids. *Gastroenterology* 1990;99:1134-1139.

[9] Camisasca M, Crosignani A, Baltezzati PM, Albisetti W, Grandinetti G, Pietrogrande L, Biffi A, Zuin M, Podda M. Parenteral calcitonin for metabolic bone disease associated with primary biliary cirrhosis. *Hepatology* 1994;20:633-637.

[10] Pares A, Guañabens N. Osteoporosis in primary biliary cirrhosis: pathogenesis and treatment. *Clin Liver Dis* 2008;(12):407-424.

[11] Gallego-Rojo FJ, Gonzalez-Calvin JL, Munoz-Torres M, Mundi JL, Fernandez-Perez R, Rodrigo-Moreno D. Bone mineral density, serum insulin-like growth factor I, and bone turnover markers in viral cirrhosis. *Hepatology* 1998;28:695-699.

[12]   Monegal A, Navasa M, Guañabens N, Peris P, Pons F, Martínez de Osaba MJ, Rimola A, Rodés J, Muñoz-Gomez J. Osteoporosis and bone mineral metabolism disorders in cirrhotic patients referred for orthotopic liver transplantation. *Calcif Tissue Int* 1997;60:148-154.

[13]   Crawford BAL, Kam C, Donaghy AJ, McCaughan GW. The heterogeneity of bone disease in cirrhosis: a multivariate analysis. *Osteoporos Int* 2003;14:987-994.

[14]   Goral V, Simsek M, Mete N. Hepatic osteodystrophy and liver cirrhosis. *World J Gastroenterol* 2010;16:1639-1643.

[15]   Malik P, Gasser RW, Kemmler G, Moncayo R, Finkenstedt G, Kurz M, Fleischhaker WW. Low bone mineral density and impaired bone metabolism in young alcoholic patients without liver cirrhosis: a cross-sectional study. *Alcohol Clin Exp Res* 2009;33(2):375-381.

[16]   Kim MJ, Shim MS, Kim MK, Lee Y, Shin YG, Chung CH, Kwon SO. Effect of chronic alcohol ingestion on bone mineral density in males without liver cirrhosis. *Korean J Inter Med* 2011;18:174-180.

[17]   Gonzalez-Calvin JL, García-Sanchez A, Bellot V, Muñoz-Torres M, Raya-Alvarez E, Salvatierra-Ríos D. Mineral metabolism, osteoblastic function and bone mass in chronic alcoholism. *Alcohol Alcohol* 1993;28:571-579.

[18]   Laitinen K, Karkkainen M, Lalla M, Lamberg-Allardt C, Tunninen R, Tahtela R, Valimaki M. Is alcohol an osteoporosis-inducing agent for young and middle-age women?. *Metabolism* 1993;42:875-881.

[19]   Schiefke I, Fach A, Wiedmann M, Aretin AV, Schenker E, Borte G, Wiese M, Moessner J. Reduced bone mineral density and altered bone turnover markers in patients with non-cirrhotic chronic hepatitis B or C infection. *World J Gastroenterol* 2005;11:1843-1847.

[20]   Diamond T, Stiel D, Lunzer M, Wilkinson M, Roche J, Posen S. Osteoporosis and skeletal fractures in chronic liver disease. *Gut* 1990;31:82-87.

[21]   George J, Ganesh HK, Acharya S, Bandgar TR, Shivane V, Karvat A, Bhatia SJ, Shah S, Menon PS, Shah N. Bone mineral density and disorders of mineral metabolism in chronic liver disease. *World J Gastroenterol* 2009;15:3516-3522.

[22]   Nanda KS, Ryan EJ, Murray BF, Brady JJ, McKenna MJ, Nolan N, O'Farrelly C, Hegarty JE. Effect of chronic hepatitis C virus infection on bone disease in postmenopausal women. *Clin Gastroenterol Hepatol* 2009;7:894-899.

[23] Raslan HM, Elhosary Y, Ezzat WM, Rasheed EA, Rasheed MA. The potential role of insulin-like growth factor 1, insulin-like growth factor binding protein 3 and bone mineral density in patients with chronic hepatitis C virus in Cairo, Egypt. *Trans R Soc Trop Med Hyg* 2010;104:429-432.

[24] Collier JD, Ninkovic M, Compston JE. Guidelines on the management of osteoporosis associated with chronic liver disease. *Gut* 2002;50(Suppl I):i1-i9.

[25] Angulo P, Therneau TM, Jogensen RA, De Sotel CK, Egan KS, Dickson ER, Hay JE, Lindor KD. Bone disease in patients with primary sclerosing cholangitis: prevalence, severity and prediction of progression. *J Hepatol* 1998;29:729-735.

[26] Diamond T, Stiel D, Posen S. Osteoporosis in hemocromatosis: iron excess, gonadal defficiency, or other factors? *Ann Intern Med* 1989;110:430-436.

[27] Sanchez AJ, Aranda-Michel J. Liver disease and osteoporosis. *Nutr Clin Pract* 2006;21:273-278.

[28] Crosbie OM, Freaney R, McKenna MJ, Hegarty JE. Bone density, vitamin D status, and disordered bone remodeling in end-stage chronic liver disease. *Calcif Tissue Int* 1999;64:295-300.

[29] Duarte MP, Farias ML, Coelho HS, Mendonca LM, Stabnov LM, do C, Lamy RA, Oliveira DS. Calcium-parathyroid hormone-vitamin D axis and metabolic bone disease in chronic viral liver disease. *J Gastroenterol Hepatol* 2001;16:1022-1027.

[30] Arteh J, Narra S, Nair S. Prevalence of vitamin D deficiency in chronic liver disease. *Dig Dis Sci* 2010;55:2624-2628.

[31] Crawford BA, Labio ED, Strasser SI, McCaughan GW. Vitamin D replacement for cirrhosis-related bone disease. *Nat Clin Pract Gastroenterol Hepatol* 2006;3:689-699.

[32] Hay JE. Osteoporosis in liver diseases and after liver transplantation. *J Hepatol* 2003;83:856-865.

[33] Pereira FA, Facincani I, Jorgetti V, Ramalho LN, Volpon JB, Dos Reis LM, de Paula FJ. Etiopathogenesis of hepatic osteodystrophy in Wistar rats with cholestatic liver disease. *Calcif Tissue Int* 2009;85:75-83.

[34] Szalay F, Hegedus D, Lakatos PL, Tornai I, Bajnok E, Dunkel K, Lakatos P. High serum osteoprotegerin and low RANKL in primary biliary cirrhosis. *J Hepatol* 2003;38:395-400.

[35] Moschen AR, Kaser A, Stadlmann S, Millonig G, Kaser S, Mühlechner P, Habior A, Graziadei I, Vogel V, Tilg H. The RANKL/OPG system

and bone mineral density in patients with chronic liver disease. *J Hepatol* 2005;43:973-983.

[36] Gonzalez-Calvin JL, Mundi JL, Casado-Caballero FJ, Abadia AC, Martin-Ibañez JJ. bone mineral density and serum levels of soluble tumor necrosis factors, estradiol, and osteoprotegerin in postmenopausal women with cirrhosis after viral hepatitis. *J Clin Metab* 2009;94:4844-4850.

[37] Olivier BJ, Schoenmaker T, Mebius RE, Everts V, Mulder CJ, van Nieuwkerk KM, de Vries TJ, van der Merwe SW. Increased osteoclast formation and activity by peripheral blood mononuclear cells in chronic liver disease patients with osteopenia. *Hepatology* 2008;47:259-267.

[38] Bell H, Raknerud N, Falch JA, Haug E. Inappropriately low levels of gonadotrophins in amenorrhoeic women with alcoholic and non-alcoholic cirrhosis. *Eur J Endocrinol* 1995;132:444-449.

[39] Garcia-Valdecasas-Campelo E, Gonzalez-Reimers E, Santolaria-Fernandez F, De la Vega-Prieto MJ, Milena-Abril A, Sanchez-Perez MJ, Martinez-Riera A, Gomez-Rodriguez MDLA. Serum osteoprotegerin and RANKL levels in chronic alcoholic liver disease. *Alcohol Alcoholism* 2006;41:261-266.

[40] Janes CH, Dickinson ER, Okazaki R, Bonde S, McDonagh AF, Riggs BL. Role of hyperbilirubinemia in the impairment of osteoblast proliferation associated with cholestatic jaundice. *J Clin Invest* 1995;95:2581-2586.

[41] Weinreb M, Pollak RD, Ackerman Z. Experimental cholestatic liver disease through bile-duct ligation in rats results in skeletal fragility and impaired osteoblastogenesis. *J Hepatol* 2004;40:385-390.

[42] Menon K, Angulo P, Weston S, Dickson ER, Lindor K. bone disease in primary biliary cirrhosis:independent indicators and rate of progression. *J Hepatol* 2001;35:316-323.

[43] Smith DL, Shire NJ, Watts NB, Schmitter T, Szabo G, Zucker SD. Hyperbilirubinemia is not a major contributing factor to altered bone mineral density in patients with chronic liver disease. *J Clin Densitom* 2006;9:105-113.

[44] Pares A, Guañabens N, Rodés J. Gene polymorphisms as predictors of decreased bone mineral density and osteoporosis in primary biliary cirrhosis. *Eur J Gastroenterol Hepatol* 2005;17:311-315.

[45] Lakatos PL, Bajnok E, Tornai I, Folhoffer A, Horwath A, Lakatos P, Habior A, Szalay F. *Insulin-like growth factor I gene microsatellite*

repeat, collagen type Ialpha1 gene Sp1 polymorphism, and bone disease in primary biliary cirrhosis. 2004;16:753-759.

[46] Hay JE, Guichelaar MMJ. Evaluation and management of osteoporosis in liver disease. *Clin Liver Dis* 2005;9:747-766.

[47] Crippin JS, Jorgensen RA, Dickson ER, Lindor KD. Hepatic osteodystrophy in primary biliary cirrhosis: effects of medical treatment. *Am J Gastroenterol* 1994;89:47-50.

[48] Carey EJ, Balan V, Kremers WK, Hay JE. Osteopenia and osteoporosis in patients with end-stage liver disease caused by hepatitis C and alcoholic liver disease: not just a cholestatic problem. *Liver Transpl* 2003;9:1166-1173.

[49] Luchi S, Fiorini I, Meini M, Scasso A. Alterations of bone metabolism in patients with chronic C virus hepatitis. *Infez Med* 2005;13:23-27.

[50] Jablkowski M, Bialkowska J, Bartkowiak J, Zygmunt A, Kurnatowska I, Nowicki M, Lewinski A. Evaluation of bone mineral density in women with chronic liver diseases during perimenopausal period. *Pol Arch Med Wewn* 2006;116:924-929.

[51]   AGA Technical review on osteoporosis in hepatic disorders. *Gastroenterology* 2003;125:941-966.

[52] Yenice N, Gumrah M, Mehtap O, Kozan A, Turkmen S. Assessment of bone metabolism and mineral density in chronic viral hepatitis. *Turk J Gastroenterol* 2006;17:260-266.

[53] Wariaghli G, Mounach A, Achemlal L, Benbaghdadi I, Aouragh A, Bezza A, El Maghraoui A. Osteoporosis in chronic liver disease: a case-control study. *Rheumatol Int* 2010;30:893-899.

[54] Arase Y, Suzuki F, Suzuki Y, Akuta N, Kobayashi M, Kawamura Y, Yatsuji H, Sezaki H, Hosaka T, Ikeda K, Kumada H. Prolonged-efficacy of bisphosphonate in postmenopausal women with osteoporosis and chronic liver disease. *J Med Virol* 2008;80:1302-1307.

[55] Guañabens N, Pares A, Ros I, Alvarez L, Pons F, Caballeria L, Monegal A, Martínez de Osaba MJ, Roca M, Peris P, Rodés J. Alendronate is more effective than etidronate for increasing bone mass in osteopenic patients with primary biliary cirrhosis. *Am J Gastroenterol* 2003;98:2268-2274.

[56] Zein CO, Jorgensen RA, Clarke B, Wenger D, Keach JC, Angulo P, Lindor KD. Alendronate improves bone mineral density in primary biliary cirrhosis: a randomized placebo-controlled trial. *Hepatology* 2005;42:762-771.

[57] Behre HM, von Eckardstein S, Kliesch S, Nieschlag E. Long-term substitution therapy of hypogonadal men with transscrotal testosterone over 7-10 years. *Clin Endocrinol* 1999;50:629-635.

[58] O´Donohue J, Williams J. Hormone replacement therapy in women with liver disease. *B J Obstet Gynaecol* 1997;104:1-3.

[59] Selby PL, Peacock M. The effect of transdermal oestrogen on bone, calcium regulating hormones and liver in postmenopausal women. *Clin Endocrinol Oxf* 1986;25:543-547.

[60] American College of Obstetricians and Gynecologists. Statement on results of the HERS II trial on hormone replacement therapy. *Gynecol Obstet Mex* 2002;70:406-408.

[61] Writing Group for the Women´s Health Initiative Investigators. Risks and benefits of estrogen plus progestin in healthy postmenopausal women. Principal results from the Women´s Health Initiative randomized controlled trial. *JAMA* 2002;288:321-333.

[62] Levy C, Harnois DM, Angulo P, Jorgensen R, Lindor. Raloxifene improves bone mass in osteopenic woman with primary biliary cirrhosis: results of a pilot study. *Liver Int* 2005;25:117-121.

[63] Dresner-Pollak R, Gabet Y, Steimatzky A, Hamdani G, Bab I, Ackerman Z, Weinreb M. Human parathyroid hormone 1-34 prevents bone loss in experimental biliary cirrhosis in rats. *Gastroenterology* 2008;134:259-267.

[64] European Association for the Study of the Liver. EASL Clinical Practice Guidelines: Management of hepatitis C virus infection. *J Hepatol* 2011;55:245-264.

[65] Solis-Herruzo JA, Castellano G, Fernandez I, Munoz R, Hawkins F. Decreased bone mineral density after therapy with alpha interferon in combination with ribavirin for chronic hepatitis C. *J Hepatol* 2000;33:812-817.

[66] Moreira RO, Balduino A, Martins HS, Reis JS, Duarte ME, Farias ML, Borojevic R. Ribavirin, but not interferon alpha-2b, is associated with impaired osteoblast proliferation and differentiation in vitro. *Calcif Tissue Int* 2004;75:160-168.

[67] Lee J, Kim JH, Kim K, Jin HM, Lee KB, Chung DJ, Kim N. Ribavirin enhances osteoclast formation through osteoblasts via up-regulation of TRANCE/RANKL. *Mol Cell Biochem* 2007;296:17-24.

[68] Trombetti A, Giostra E, Mentha G, Negro F, Rizzoli R. Lack of evidence for ribavirin-induced bone loss. *Hepatology* 2002;36:255-257.

[69] Hofmann WP, Kronenberger B, Bojunga J, Stamm B, Herrmann E, Bucker A, Mihm U, von WM, Zeuzem S, Sarrazin C. Prospective study of bone mineral density and metabolism in patients with chronic hepatitis C during pegylated interferon alpha and ribavirin therapy. *J Viral Hepat* 2008;15:790-796.

[70] Arase Y, Suzuki F, Suzuki Y, Akuta N, Kobayashi M, Sezaki H, Hosaka T, Kawamura Y, Yatsuji H, Hirakawa M, Ikeda K, Hsieh SD, Oomoto Y, Amakawa K, Kato H, Kazawa T, Tsuji H, Kobayashi T, Kumada H. Virus clearance reduces bone fracture in postmenopausal women with osteoporosis and chronic liver disease caused by hepatitis C virus. *J Med Virol* 2010;82:390-395.

[71] Crosbie OM, Freaney R, McKenna MJ, Curry MP, Hegarty JE. Predicting bone loss following orthotopic liver transplantation. *Gut* 1999;44:430-434.

[72] Negri AL, Plantalech LC, Russo Picasso MF, Otero A, Sarli M. Post-transplantation osteoporosis. *Medicina (B Aires)* 1999;59:777-786.

[73] Hamburg SM, Piers DA, van den Berg AP, Slooff MJ, Haagsma EB. Bone mineral density in the long term after liver transplantation. *Osteoporos Int* 2000;11:600-606.

[74] Crosbie OM, Freaney R, McKenna MJ, Curry MP, Hegarty JE. Predicting bone loss following orthotopic liver transplantation. *Gut* 1999;44:430-434.

[75] Porayko MK, Wiesner RH, Hay JE. Bone disease in liver transplant recipients: incidence, timing and risk factors. *Transplant Proc* 1991;23:1462-1465.

[76] McDonald JA, Dunstan CR, Dilworth P. Bone loss after liver transplantation. *Hepatology* 1991;14:613-619.

[77] Eastell R, Dickson ER, Hodgson SF. Rates of vertebral bone loss before and after liver transplantation in women with primary biliary cirrhosis. *Hepatology* 1991;14:296-300.

[78] Guichelaar MMJ, Kendall R, Malinchoc M, Hay JE. Bone mineral density before and after OLT: long-term follow-up and predictive factors. *Liver Transpl.* 2005;12:1390-1402.

[79] Cunningham J. Posttransplantation bone disease. *Transplantation* 2005;79:629-634.

[80] Millonig G, Graziadei I, Eichler D, Pfeiffer KP, Finkenstedt G, Muehllechner P, Koenigsrainer A, Margreiter R, Vogel W. Alendronate in combination with calcium and vitamin D prevents bone loss after

orthotopic liver transplantation: a prospective single-center study. *Liver Transpl* 2005;11:960-966.

[81] Crawford BAL, Kam C, Pavlovic J, Byth K, Handelsman DJ, Angus PW, McCaughan GW. Zoledronic acid prevents bone loss after liver transplantation: a randomized, double-blind, placebo-controlled trial. *Ann Inter Med* 2006;144:239-248.

[82] Valero MA, Loinaz C, Larrodera L. Calcitonin and bisphosphonates treatment in bone loss after liver transplantation. *Calcif Tissue Int* 1995;57:15-19.

In: Hepatitis C Virus
Editors: A. P. Gonzales et al.

ISBN 978-1-61942-674-0
© 2012 Nova Science Publishers, Inc.

Chapter IV

SOCS1 Involvement in Liver Damage during Hepatitis C Virus Infection

Virginia Sedeño-Monge[1,2], Francisca Sosa-Jurado[1],
Verónica Vallejo-Ruiz[1], Gerardo Santos-López[1]
and Julio Reyes-Leyva[1]*
[1]Laboratorio de Biología Molecular y Virología,
Centro de Investigación Biomédica de Oriente, Instituto Mexicano del
Seguro Social, Metepec, Puebla, México
[2]Facultad de Medicina, Universidad Popular Autónoma del Estado de
Puebla, Puebla, México

ABSTRACT

Hepatitis C virus (HCV) is a public health concern worldwide and a
major cause of hepatic cirrhosis and hepatocellular carcinoma (HCC).
Current therapy for HCV infection is the administration of pegylated-
interferon-alpha (IFN-α) plus ribavirin; however, ~50% of treated
patients do not respond to interferon therapy and, thus, are not able to
clear virus infection. IFN-α plays a pivotal role in the response against

* Facultad de Medicina, Universidad Popular Autónoma del Estado de Puebla, 21 sur 1103 CP
72410 Puebla, México E-mail: virginia.sedeno@upaep.mx, vikysm@hotmail.com.

viral infections, acting through its specific cell receptors that activate the JAK-STAT signaling pathway and inducing the expression of hundreds of genes that code for proteins with antiviral functions. The antiviral activity generated by interferon is negatively controlled by several proteins, among them the suppressor of cytokine signaling 1 (SOCS1), which is a negative regulator of the JAK-STAT signaling pathway induced by different cytokines (IFNα/β, IFNγ, IL-6 and IL-4). *Socs1* deficiency is associated with chronic liver alterations. Diploid knockout mice (SOCS1$^{-/-}$) presented fatty degeneration and hepatic necrosis, whereas haploid elimination (SOCS1$^{-/+}$) increased progression to hepatic fibrosis. In addition, silencing of s*ocs1* gene by methylation induced a permanent activation of the JAK-STAT pathway in HCC cell lines, suggesting that *socs1* is a tumor suppressor. In this chapter we review the participation of *socs1* in several molecular mechanisms involved in liver damage during HCV infection.

INTRODUCTION

Cytokines are proteins that participate in many biological processes including immunity, healing and hematopoiesis. Cellular response induced by cytokines depends on the type of stimulatory molecule and the target cell, produced as a result of cellular function, proliferation, differentiation, activation or inhibition [1]. The imbalance in cytokine synthesis or activity is involved in adverse processes in the human body such as malignant transformation and immune pathologies, i.e., autoimmunity and allergy [2].

Cytokines are recognized by four different classes of receptors and use similar transduction signals to carry out their functions [3]. Interaction between a cytokine and its receptor induces dimerization of the specific receptor subunits and activation of Janus kinase (JAK) that phosphorylates tyrosine residues in the cytoplasmic domain of the receptors and creates recruiting points for signal transducers and activators of transcription (STAT). When STAT proteins are phosphorylated, they form homo- or heterodimers. STAT dimers associate with a third component called IRF9 (interferon response factor 9) or p48 that allows them to migrate into the nucleus and associate with specific response elements at promoter regions of several genes inducing their transcription.

Three families of negative regulators induced by cytokines have been identified: a) SHP2 phosphatases, which are constitutively expressed and dephosphorylate JAK kinases and cytokine receptors; b) protein inhibitors of activated STAT (PIAS) that also are constitutively expressed [4]; and c) suppressor of cytokine signalling (SOCS) that are stimulated by elements of the activated signaling pathway induced by cytokines [5] (Figure 1).

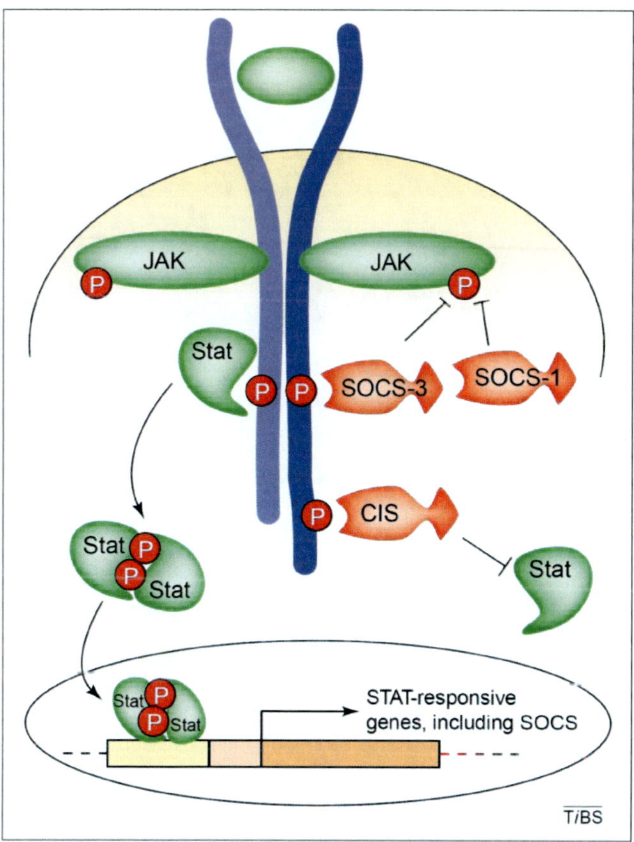

Figure 1. Cytokine signal transduction and signal attenuation by SOCS proteins (From Kile BT *et al.*, *Trends Biochem Sci* 2002, 27:235-24. With permission from Elsevier).

THE SOCS FAMILY

The SOCS protein family is comprised of eight members: SOCS1 to SOCS7 and the cytokine-inducible SH2-containing (CIS) protein [6]. Proteins and mRNA of SOCS1, SOCS2, SOCS3 and CIS are generally present at low levels in non-stimulated cells, possibly due to their repressive action. The expression of SOCS is quickly stimulated in response to cytokines, and STAT proteins play an important role in inducing transcription of these genes. SOCS1 and SOCS3 are powerful inhibitors of the signals induced by cytokines. Many pathological agents also induce the expression of SOCS proteins [7, 8].

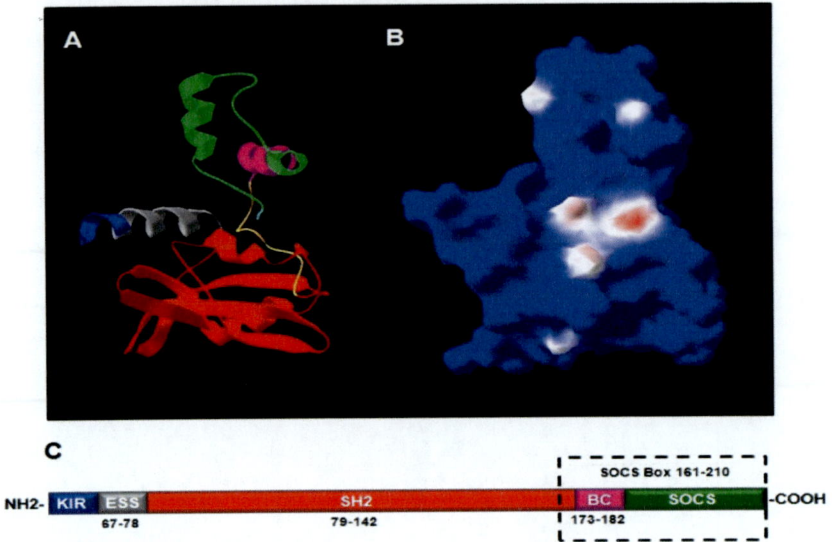

Figure 2. Structural model of SOCS1. (A-B) Tridimensional model constructed in Swiss-Prot database, using as a template the structure of crystallized SOCS2 protein (access number PDB2c9w). (C) Schematic distribution of SOCS1 functional domains; KIR inhibitory region of the kinase, ESS extended SH2 subdomain, SH2 domain, BC region interaction with B and C elongins. The distinction of the domains in the tridimensional model A was realized using the same colours as in (C).

STRUCTURE OF SOCS PROTEINS

Members of the SOCS family present a central portion with a SH2 domain formed by 96 amino acids and organized in six or seven β-sheets surrounded by two α-helices. The SH2 domain works as a regulator of the intracellular signaling cascades, interacting with high affinity to phosphotyrosine-containing target peptides in a sequence-specific manner. The phosphotyrosine in the phosphopeptide inserts into a positively charged pocket in the SH2 domain located on the N-terminal side of the central β-sheet [9]. SH2 domain is flanked in the N-terminal by a variable length fragment including a kinase inhibitory region (KIR) and an extended SH2 subdomain (12 amino acids each). The SOCS box is a domain of 40-50 amino acids found in some protein families that inhibit kinases through ubiquitination mediated by elongins. SOCS box is constituted by two blocks of conserved residues separated by two to ten non-conserved residues; the C-terminus is rich in leucine and proline and the BC region binds to B and C elongins [10, 11]. A protein structure model is shown in Figure 2.

SOCS1

SOCS1, also known as JAB (JAK-binding protein) and SSI (STAT-induced STAT inhibitor-1), is codified by *socs1* gene located in chromosome 16p13.13 downstream of the protamine genes cluster and within a CpG island (a region rich in cytokine and guanine). *Socs1* has an extension of 2.5 kb and contains two exons codifying a protein of 211 amino acids [12-14].

THE BIOLOGICAL FUNCTION OF SOCS1

Several cytokines such as IL-6, IL-4, IL-3, IFN-γ and granulocyte-macrophage colony stimulating factor (GM-SCF) induce *socs1* expression in hematopoietic cells, which acts as a negative feedback regulator to inhibit the biologic effects of these cytokines [12, 14]. Increase in expression of *socs1* modifies the signals induced by IFN-α/β, widely abolishing their pro-apoptotic effects [15]. SOCS1 also suppresses signals induced by IL-4 and IFN-γ, maintaining the balance between favorable immunological activities and pathological effects due to overexpression of these cytokines [16].

SOCS1 is normally expressed in mouse thymocytes and inhibits cytokine signaling involved in differentiation and maturation of T lymphocytes, suggesting that abnormalities in mice lacking this protein may result in altered immune responses. SOCS1 regulates T-cell differentiation and completes signals initiated by IFN-γ in lymphoid and non-lymphoid cells to control the production of inflammatory cytokines such as TNF-α.

It has been established that the lethality associated with SOCS1 deficiency in mice models requires the presence of T lymphocytes due to the increased serum levels of IFN-γ, which are produced mainly by these cells. Altered differentiation or regulation of T cells in SOCS1-deficient mice leads to increased production of IFN-γ [17].

SOCS1 modulates signals involved in the innate response against virus infections, including the activation pathways for IFN-α, IFNAR/JAK-STAT and TLR/RIG-1 (Toll-like receptors/retinoic acid-inducible gene 1) [18]. Inhibition of the antiviral state depends on three mechanisms involving SOCS1 protein: 1) modulation of JAK activity, 2) competence with STAT proteins for IFNAR binding sites, and 3) ubiquitination and subsequent degradation by the ubiquitin-proteasome complex [19]. This regulatory pathway is manifested broadly in cells infected by many pathogens such as hepatitis C virus (HCV), respiratory syncytial virus, Newcastle disease virus, Sendai virus, vesicular stomatitis virus, etc.

In all these cases, type I IFN-α/β secretion is induced when the TLR/RIG-1 route is activated [20, 21]. Indeed, the presence of viral proteins and nucleic acids is recognized by TLRs and RIG-1 sensors that initiate the innate and adaptive immune responses; these molecules also induce the expression of SOCS [19].

SOCS1 inhibits type I IFN signaling through an interaction with IFNAR1-associated kinase, Tyk2, with the KIR domain being essential in this action. Analysis of IFNAR1 internalisation has shown a role for SOCS1 in controlling IFNAR1 surface expression following IFN-α signaling. Although there were not significant baseline differences, the process internalisation/recycling of IFNAR1 was reduced in cells lacking SOCS1 [22].

Another effect of JAK-STAT pathway inhibition induced by SOCS1 is the blocking of feedback signals that ensure the establishment of a robust innate immunity. In this regard, recognition of pathogen-associated molecular patterns by TLR/RIG1 is conducive to activation of IRF7 and IRF3, which amplify IFN-α and IFN-β gene transcription.

Expression of IRF7 depends on the functionality of the JAK-STAT pathway because IRF7 is an interferon-stimulated gene (ISG); therefore, its inhibition by SOCS1 indirectly reduces the potential of IRF7 to activate the antiviral response. It has been shown that SOCS1 indirectly suppresses the effects of the signals induced by double-stranded RNA generated during viral infection and negatively regulates the antiviral immune response to avoid overreaction [23].

It has also been reported that SOCS1-transfected cells show a marked increase in the expression of NF-κB and IL-8 genes, which are key molecules in the activation of inflammatory responses. IL-8 is a chemokine that induces migration, adhesion and degranulation of neutrophils; whereas NF-κB is a nuclear factor that forms a complex with IRF3 on the promoter of IFN-β gene inducing its transcription [19].

SOCS1 EXPRESSION DURING HEPATITIS C VIRUS INFECTION

HCV is responsible for chronic processes of the liver such as cirrhosis and hepatocellular carcinoma (HCC). The treatment of choice for chronic HCV infection is combined therapy of pegylated IFN-α plus ribavirin. However, 50% of patients infected with HCV 1b genotype do not achieve an improvement in health. Some viral proteins including NS5A, C and E2 have been implicated in the pathogenesis of liver infection and evasion of antiviral response induced by IFN-α. NS5A protein possesses a structural domain referred to as interferon sensitivity-determining region (ISDR) that binds and inhibits RNA-dependent protein kinase (PKR), an antiviral protein generated in response to IFN-α [24]. The structural E2 protein contains a sequence of 12 amino acids that possesses a high degree of similarity with the phosphorylation sites for PKR. Through this interaction, E2 functions as a false substrate inhibiting antiviral functions of PKR [25].

The levels of *socs1* mRNA in liver of patients with HCV are significantly lower than in patients without infection. This is important because SOCS1 possesses a tumor suppressor activity, thus, its reduction may contribute to liver carcinogenesis associated with HCV infection. In this regard, expression of HCV core protein in mice that develop HCC suppresses the expression of *socs1* and *irf-1* mRNA after stimulation with IL-6. With regard to the methylation status of the *socs1* gene, no hypermethylation was observed in the *socs1* gene of the core gene transgenic mice either at the 5′-noncoding region or the CpG island at the coding region [26].

The reduction of STAT3 phosphorylation (a transcription factor for *socs1*) induced by HCV core protein may be implicated in *socs1* suppression. However, transport and activation of STAT1 to nucleus are not interrupted due to core protein, but affect the expression of STAT target genes IRF-1, c-myc and bcl-X_L. When the cells are stimulated with IL-6, IRF-1 decreases, c-myc is unaffected and bcl-X_L is increased. These results suggest that STAT activation is deteriorated by the expression of HCV core protein; however, the precise role of this protein in suppression of *socs1* has not been defined [26].

Socs3 and *socs1* overexpression diminish IFN-α signaling and expression of antiviral proteins MxA and 2′5 OAS in hepatic cells. This mechanism has been implicated in the resistance to the treatment with IFN-α in patients infected with HCV [27]. There is evidence that HCV may affect the signaling of JAK-STAT pathway [28, 29]. Expression of *socs1* in the liver of patients infected with HCV seems to be implicated in the resistance to treatment with IFN-α and IFN-λ. *Socs1* transcription seems to increase in patients with chronic HCV treated with IFN-α and ribavirin with regard to patients without therapy. This suggests that *socs1* transcription depends more on IFN signaling pathway than on induction by HCV infection. Patients infected with HCV genotypes 1a and 1b present higher transcription levels of *socs1* than other genotypes [30].

Additionally, an inhibitory effect of *socs1* has been found on IL-10 signaling [31]. SOCS1 can suppress IFN-induced phosphorylation of STAT and expression of antiviral proteins 2′,5′ OAS and MxA in human hepatoma cells. This mechanism may contribute to the putative role of SOCS proteins in the IFN resistance in HCV infection [32].

ROLE OF SOCS1 IN LIVER STEATOSIS

Hepatic steatosis is the accumulation of fat vacuoles in the cytoplasm of hepatocytes. The causes implicated in the pathogenesis of hepatic steatosis correlate with the presence of concomitant infections, obesity, drug abuse, dyslipidemia, alcohol intake and type 2 diabetes mellitus, in addition to non-alcoholic steatohepatitis (NASH) [32]. Liver steatosis is a common histopathological finding in patients with chronic hepatitis C. A significant proportion of these patients have fatty liver, suggesting the possibility of a direct cytopathic effect of HCV when other non-viral risk factors have been excluded [33].

Sterol regulatory element binding protein (SREBP)-1 is a key regulator of fatty acid synthesis in the liver. STAT3 and STAT5b show inhibitory effects on *srebp-1* promoter activity in mice induced to express *socs1*. An increased expression of SREBP-1 has been observed, possibly due to suppression of STAT3 phosphorylation by SOCS1. Therefore, SOCS1 induced the increment of both SREBP-1 expression and fatty acid synthesis in the liver [34].

INACTIVATION OF SOCS1
AND INDUCTION OF FIBROSIS

Liver fibrosis is a result of the inflammatory process and tissue repair in response to prolonged liver damage and is characterized by the accumulation of connective tissue due to a significant disproportion between production and degradation of the extracellular matrix. During the process of fibrosis generation, stellate cells are transformed into myofibroblasts that produce types I and III collagen; meanwhile, Kupffer cells stimulate stellate cells by means of TGF-β for the secretion of extracellular matrix components [35].

It has been observed that chemical induction of fibrosis in SOCS1 haploid-deficient mice induces fatty degeneration in hepatocytes, activation and proliferation of hepatic stellate cells, macrophage infiltration, *socs1* mRNA reduction and increased levels of IL-6, TGF-β and IFN-β. In addition, fibrotic tissue also presented activation of STAT1, reduced activation of STAT3, and a significant increase of IRF-1 [36]. These results indicate that SOCS1 deficiency is inversely proportional to liver fibrosis.

Recent evidence indicates that members of the platelet-derived growth factor (PDFG) family are also important factors in the development of liver fibrosis [37-40] because transgenic mice with liver-specific overexpression of PDFG-B or PDFG-C rapidly develop liver fibrosis [37]. PDFG is closely associated with the transcriptional induction of TGFB; both factors act through activation of STAT. It is believed that the pro-fibrogenic activity of PDFGs and TGFB is associated with activation of hepatic stellate cells and advancement of liver fibrosis to HCC.

A significant decrease of activated forms of STAT1 and STAT3 is associated with development of liver fibrosis at early pre-neoplastic stages of hepatocarcinogenesis followed by a marked upregulation of STAT3 in the fully developed HCC. *Socs1* expression is increased in the early stages of liver fibrosis; however, progression to HCC is characterized by an inhibition of *socs1* gene expression.

Meanwhile, increase in the c-Myc and cyclin D1 protein levels in HCC is associated with STAT3 activation. The opposing trends between *socs1* expression and STAT3 activation levels suggest that SOCS1 acts as a potent negative-feedback inhibitor of STAT3.

This suggests that during early stages of neoplastic cell transformation, overexpression of *socs1* effectively inhibits TGFB and PDFG-induced STAT3 activation and the consequent upregulation of known downstream inducers of cell proliferation such as cyclin d1 and c-Myc genes. During the advanced stages of carcinogenesis, *socs1* downregulation results in loss of its ability to attenuate the signals from the upregulated TGFB and PDFG, leading to oncogenic STAT3 activation and malignant cell transformation. Downregulation of *socs1* expression may be a crucial event in the transformation process leading to [41].

ROLE OF SOCS1
IN THE CONTROL OF CARCINOGENESIS

The main causes of HCC are hepatitis B virus, HCV, aflatoxin B (a mycotoxin), alcohol, hemochromatosis with low risk, α-1 antitrypsin deficiency, tyrosinemia, etc. It is estimated that hepatitis B and C viruses represent the main risk [42]. HCC usually develops after one or more decades of suffering from HCV infection and the risk is restricted to patients with cirrhosis or advanced fibrosis. Although HCV-infected patients with mild fibrosis are not candidates to develop HCC, once cirrhosis is established, HCC develops at an incidence of 1-4% per year and there is a strong correlation between fibrosis and development of HCC [43].

SOCS1 is activated and blocks JAK activation, leading to signal attenuation or termination in normal cells. However, in some cancers cells, *socs1* gene is silenced by methylation, leaving permanent activation of the JAK-STAT pathway. As a result, tumor cells have no control over cell growth. The JAK-STAT route is persistently activated in various transformed tissues, which has been implicated in promotion of cancer. For example, JAK2 is activated in B-cell leukemias; JAK1, JAK3, STAT3 and STAT5 in T cells infected by lymphotropic virus HTLV-1; JAK1 and JAK3 in pre-B cells transformed by the oncogene *v-abl* of murine leukemia of Abelson; STAT1 and STAT3 in acute myeloid leukemia and Burkitt lymphoma; STAT3 in mouse-transformed fibroblasts and in cell lines of human breast carcinoma activated by *v-src*, *v-fps* and *v-sis* oncogenes [44].

SOCS1 SILENCING AND HCC

Between 50% and 60% of the human gene promoters have a high density of control regions known as CpG islands. These regions regulate a large number of constituent genes, oncogenes and tumor suppressor genes. In the remainder of the genome there is an average of 70% to 80% of CpG islands, which are mostly methylated [45].

The process of methylation is involved in irreversible silencing of genes during different stages of development. At birth, this process contributes to switching-off of embryonic genes that will not be expressed during the adult stage. However, methylation is also an epigenetic modification that can lead to tumor processes. Modification of CpG islands is carried out by the addition of a methyl group to carbon 5 of cytosine by DNA methyltransferase enzymes [46]. Among the abnormal or aberrant methylated genes are some tumor suppressor genes such as *Rb* (retinoblastoma) and *p16INK4a* (an inhibitor of cyclin-dependent kinases) [45]. A family of proteins that bind to DNA known as methyl-binding proteins (MBD) has been identified. These interact with methylated DNA and, with the help of co-repressors, initiate the remodeling of chromatin, inducing a more compact form due to the action of histone acetylase [47].

It has been found that 65% of 26 human primary HCC tumor samples show aberrant methylation in *socs1* CpG islands and silencing of its transcription [44]. In cells with methylated *socs1* gene, binding of DNA to the nuclear matrix is reduced, suggesting that DNA methylation facilitates dynamic changes in the chromatin structure. The high incidence of *socs1* gene inactivation by methylation suggests a pathophysiological role of *socs1* silencing in the development of HCC. Specific factors activated by JAK-STAT pathway that are responsible for oncogenesis have not been identified in the liver, but several cytokines, hormones and growth factors that stimulate this signaling pathway have been identified.

A study of the methylation pattern of *socs1* in patients infected with HCV reported that the proportion of *socs1* methylation increased significantly with the progression of fibrosis. It has been shown that severe liver fibrosis due to chronic liver inflammation is a major cause of HCC development after HCV infection. More than 45% of liver biopsies of patients with chronic HCV infection have aberrant methylation of *socs1*. These samples presented a low level of *socs1* mRNA in comparison with non-methylated DNA samples. This indicates that DNA methylation occurs before the onset of HCC in a significant percentage of patients with viral hepatitis [44]. Another study showed that *socs1* methylation was more frequent in HCC derived from cirrhosis than in HCC not associated with previous cirrhosis [48].

Liver damage chemically induced was studied in mice carrying a heterozygous deletion of the *socs1* gene (*socs1* $^{-/+}$), founding that more severe liver damage occurred in SOCS1$^{-/+}$ mice that SOCS1$^{+/+}$ mice. It has been shown that both *socs1* haploid deficiency in mice and *socs1* silencing by methylation in humans are highly correlated with liver damage, increasing liver fibrosis and carcinogenesis. However, it is unclear how *socs1* contributes to fibrosis and hepatocarcinogenesis. Although the mechanism of aberrant gene methylation is unknown, it may be caused by increases in the novo methylation activity or by a defect of the protection mechanism against de novo methylation. It is suggested that *socs1* is epigenetically methylated as fibrosis progresses, such as occurs in the methylation of tumor suppressor gene *p16* (INK4A) during liver fibrosis [49, 50].

The development of HCC is a multistep process and the sequence of chronic hepatitis-cirrhosis-dysplastic nodule-HCC has been well established. Recently, the role of epigenetic instability has been implicated in hepatocarcinogenesis and the list of tumor suppressor genes affected by such epigenetic silencing in HCC is expanding [51-56]. An increase in the number of methylating events has also been demonstrated during the course of multistep hepatocarcinogenesis. *Socs1* and other genes were used in the study of the methylation status of low-grade dysplastic nodules (LGDN), high-grade dysplastic nodules (HGDN), and early HCC (eHCC) in hepatitis B virus (HBV)-related hepatocarcinogenesis. This study showed that methylation was more frequent in dysplastic nodules and HCC, methylation levels were significantly increased from cirrhosis to LGDN, and *Socs1* methylation gradually increased along multistep hepatocarcinogenesis. In addition, none of the CpG island loci were hypermethylated in normal livers, whereas decreased SOCS1 protein expression was seen during multistep hepatocarcinogenesis. These results suggest that the epigenetic changes occur predominantly in the earlier stages of HCC development [57].

SOCS1 and other genes as APC and RASSF1A has been used for study the methylation status in the hepatitis B virus-related human multistep hepatocarcinogenesis (founding that the methylation of SOCS1 and APC was more frequent in dysplastic nodules and early hepatocellularcarcinome and the methylation levels were significantly increased from cirrhosis to low-grade dysplastic nodule. SOCS1 methylation gradually increased along hepatocarcinogenesis (Um TM et al., 2011)

CONCLUSION

SOCS1 is an important regulator of immune response. Silencing of *socs1* has been correlated with fatty degeneration, hepatic fibrosis progression and HCC development.

Several lines of evidence support that *socs1* plays an anti-oncogenic role in the liver. Chronic infection with HCV is implicated in the reduced expression of *socs1* in liver cells and is proposed as one of the causes due to the fact that HCV produces HCC.

ACKNOWLEDGMENTS

This work was supported by Instituto Mexicano del Seguro Social under project FIS/IMSS/PROT/G10/830, and the Universidad Popular Autónoma del Estado de Puebla under project 30108-176.

REFERENCES

[1]   Oberholzer A, Oberholzer C, Moldawer LL: Cytokine signaling—regulation of the immune response in normal and critically ill states. *Crit. Care. Med.* 2000, 28:N3-12.

[2]   Nicola NA: Cytokine pleiotropy and redundancy: a view from the receptor. *Stem Cells* 1994, 12 Suppl 1:3-12; discussion 12-14.

[3]   Ihle JN, Thierfelder W, Teglund S, Stravopodis D, Wang D, Feng J, Parganas E: Signaling by the cytokine receptor superfamily. *Ann. NY Acad. Sci.* 1998, 865:1-9.

[4]   Kile BT, Schulman BA, Alexander WS, Nicola NA, Martin HM, Hilton DJ: The SOCS box: a tale of destruction and degradation. *Trends Biochem. Sci.* 2002, 27:235-241.

[5]   Wormald S, Hilton DJ: Inhibitors of cytokine signal transduction. *J. Biol. Chem.* 2004, 279:821-824.

[6]   Rakesh K, Agrawal DK: Controlling cytokine signaling by constitutive inhibitors. *Biochem. Pharmacol.* 2005, 70:649-657.

[7]   Kinjyo I, Hanada T, Inagaki-Ohara K, Mori H, Aki D, Ohishi M, Yoshida H, Kubo M, Yoshimura A: SOCS1/JAB is a negative regulator of LPS-induced macrophage activation. *Immunity* 2002, 17:583-591.

[8]   Nakagawa R, Naka T, Tsutsui H, Fujimoto M, Kimura A, Abe T, Seki E, Sato S, Takeuchi O, Takeda K, et al: SOCS-1 participates in negative regulation of LPS responses. *Immunity* 2002, 17:677-687.

[9]   Waksman G, Shoelson SE, Pant N, Cowburn D, Kuriyan J: Binding of a high affinity phosphotyrosyl peptide to the Src SH2 domain: crystal structures of the complexed and peptide-free forms. *Cell* 1993, 72: 779-790.

[10]   Hilton DJ, Richardson RT, Alexander WS, Viney EM, Willson TA, Sprigg NS, Starr R, Nicholson SE, Metcalf D, Nicola NA: Twenty

proteins containing a C-terminal SOCS box form five structural classes. *Proc. Natl. Acad. Sci. USA.* 1998, 95:114-119.

[11] Zhang JG, Farley A, Nicholson SE, Willson TA, Zugaro LM, Simpson RJ, Moritz RL, Cary D, Richardson R, Hausmann G, et al: The conserved SOCS box motif in suppressors of cytokine signaling binds to elongins B and C and may couple bound proteins to proteasomal degradation. *Proc. Natl. Acad. Sci. USA* 1999, 96:2071-2076.

[12] Starr R, Willson TA, Viney EM, Murray LJ, Rayner JR, Jenkins BJ, Gonda TJ, Alexander WS, Metcalf D, Nicola NA, Hilton DJ: A family of cytokine-inducible inhibitors of signalling. *Nature* 1997, 387: 917-921.

[13] Endo TA, Masuhara M, Yokouchi M, Suzuki R, Sakamoto H, Mitsui K, Matsumoto A, Tanimura S, Ohtsubo M, Misawa H, et al: A new protein containing an SH2 domain that inhibits JAK kinases. *Nature* 1997, 387:921-924.

[14] Naka T, Narazaki M, Hirata M, Matsumoto T, Minamoto S, Aono A, Nishimoto N, Kajita T, Taga T, Yoshizaki K, et al: Structure and function of a new STAT-induced STAT inhibitor. *Nature* 1997, 387:924-929.

[15] Zitzmann K, Brand S, De Toni EN, Baehs S, Goke B, Meinecke J, Spottl G, Meyer HH, Auernhammer CJ: SOCS1 silencing enhances antitumor activity of type I IFNs by regulating apoptosis in neuroendocrine tumor cells. *Cancer Res.* 2007, 67:5025-5032.

[16] Alexander WS, Starr R, Fenner JE, Scott CL, Handman E, Sprigg NS, Corbin JE, Cornish AL, Darwiche R, Owczarek CM, et al: SOCS1 is a critical inhibitor of interferon gamma signaling and prevents the potentially fatal neonatal actions of this cytokine. *Cell* 1999, 98:597-608.

[17] Marine JC, Topham DJ, McKay C, Wang D, Parganas E, Stravopodis D, Yoshimura A, Ihle JN: SOCS1 deficiency causes a lymphocyte-dependent perinatal lethality. *Cell.* 1999, 98:609-616.

[18] Mansell A, Smith R, Doyle SL, Gray P, Fenner JE, Crack PJ, Nicholson SE, Hilton DJ, O'Neill LA, Hertzog PJ: Suppressor of cytokine signaling 1 negatively regulates Toll-like receptor signaling by mediating Mal degradation. *Nat. Immunol.* 2006, 7:148-155.

[19] Pothlichet J, Chignard M, Si-Tahar M: Cutting edge: innate immune response triggered by influenza A virus is negatively regulated by SOCS1 and SOCS3 through a RIG-I/IFNAR1-dependent pathway. *J. Immunol.* 2008, 180:2034-2038.

[20] Kato H, Takeuchi O, Sato S, Yoneyama M, Yamamoto M, Matsui K, Uematsu S, Jung A, Kawai T, Ishii KJ, et al: Differential roles of MDA5 and RIG-I helicases in the recognition of RNA viruses. *Nature* 2006, 441:101-105.

[21] Saito T, Hirai R, Loo YM, Owen D, Johnson CL, Sinha SC, Akira S, Fujita T, Gale M, Jr.: Regulation of innate antiviral defenses through a shared repressor domain in RIG-I and LGP2. *Proc. Natl. Acad. Sci. USA* 2007, 104:582-587.

[22] Piganis RA, de Weerd NA, Gould JA, Schindler CW, Mansell A, Nicholson SE, Hertzog PJ: Suppressor of cytokine signaling (SOCS)1 inhibits type I interferon (IFN) signaling via the IFNAR1 associated tyrosine kinase Tyk2. *J. Biol. Chem.* 2011, 286(39):33811-8.

[23] Dai X, Sayama K, Yamasaki K, Tohyama M, Shirakata Y, Hanakawa Y, Tokumaru S, Yahata Y, Yang L, Yoshimura A, Hashimoto K: SOCS1-negative feedback of STAT1 activation is a key pathway in the dsRNA-induced innate immune response of human keratinocytes. *J. Invest. Dermatol.* 2006, 126:1574-1581.

[24] Polyak SJ, Gerotto M: The molecular basis for responsiveness to anti-viral therapy in hepatitis C. *Forum (Genova)* 2000, 10:46-58.

[25] Taylor DR, Tian B, Romano PR, Hinnebusch AG, Lai MM, Mathews MB: Hepatitis C virus envelope protein E2 does not inhibit PKR by simple competition with autophosphorylation sites in the RNA-binding domain. *J. Virol.* 2001, 75:1265-1273.

[26] Miyoshi H, Fujie H, Shintani Y, Tsutsumi T, Shinzawa S, Makuuchi M, Kokudo N, Matsuura Y, Suzuki T, Miyamura T, et al: Hepatitis C virus core protein exerts an inhibitory effect on suppressor of cytokine signaling (SOCS)-1 gene expression. *J. Hepatol.* 2005, 43:757-763.

[27] Vlotides G, Sorensen AS, Kopp F, Zitzmann K, Cengic N, Brand S, Zachoval R, Auernhammer CJ: SOCS-1 and SOCS-3 inhibit IFN-alpha-induced expression of the antiviral proteins 2,5-OAS and MxA. *Biochem Biophys. Res. Commun.* 2004, 320:1007-1014.

[28] Duong FH, Filipowicz M, Tripodi M, La Monica N, Heim MH: Hepatitis C virus inhibits interferon signaling through up-regulation of protein phosphatase 2A. *Gastroenterology* 2004, 126:263-277.

[29] Blindenbacher A, Duong FH, Hunziker L, Stutvoet ST, Wang X, Terracciano L, Moradpour D, Blum HE, Alonzi T, Tripodi M, et al: Expression of hepatitis c virus proteins inhibits interferon alpha signaling in the liver of transgenic mice. *Gastroenterology* 2003, 124:1465-1475.

[30] Sedeno-Monge V, Santos-Lopez G, Rocha-Gracia RC, Melendez-Mena D, Ramirez-Mata A, Vallejo-Ruiz V, Reyes-Leyva J: Quantitative analysis of interferon alpha receptor subunit 1 and suppressor of cytokine signaling 1 gene transcription in blood cells of patients with chronic hepatitis C. *Virol. J.* 2010, 7:243.

[31] Ding Y, Chen D, Tarcsafalvi A, Su R, Qin L, Bromberg JS: Suppressor of cytokine signaling 1 inhibits IL-10-mediated immune responses. *J. Immunol.* 2003, 170:1383-1391.

[32] Brand S, Zitzmann K, Dambacher J, Beigel F, Olszak T, Vlotides G, Eichhorst ST, Goke B, Diepolder H, Auernhammer CJ: SOCS-1 inhibits expression of the antiviral proteins 2',5'-OAS and MxA induced by the novel interferon-lambdas IL-28A and IL-29. *Biochem. Biophys. Res. Commun.* 2005, 331:543-548.

[33] Serfaty L, Poujol-Robert A, Carbonell N, Chazouilleres O, Poupon RE, Poupon R: Effect of the interaction between steatosis and alcohol intake on liver fibrosis progression in chronic hepatitis C. *Am. J. Gastroenterol* 2002, 97:1807-1812.

[34] Ueki K, Kondo T, Tseng YH, Kahn CR: Central role of suppressors of cytokine signaling proteins in hepatic steatosis, insulin resistance, and the metabolic syndrome in the mouse. *Proc. Natl. Acad. Sci. USA* 2004, 101:10422-10427.

[35] Treviño G VK, Vidaurri A, Fernandez L: Fibrogénesis hepática. *Investigación Ciencia* 2006, 14:35-38.

[36] Sanceau J, Hiscott J, Delattre O, Wietzerbin J: IFN-beta induces serine phosphorylation of Stat-1 in Ewing's sarcoma cells and mediates apoptosis via induction of IRF-1 and activation of caspase-7. *Oncogene* 2000, 19:3372-3383.

[37] Campbell JS, Hughes SD, Gilbertson DG, Palmer TE, Holdren MS, Haran AC, Odell MM, Bauer RL, Ren HP, Haugen HS, et al: Platelet-derived growth factor C induces liver fibrosis, steatosis, and hepatocellular carcinoma. *Proc. Natl. Acad. Sci. USA* 2005, 102: 3389-3394.

[38] Czochra P, Klopcic B, Meyer E, Herkel J, Garcia-Lazaro JF, Thieringer F, Schirmacher P, Biesterfeld S, Galle PR, Lohse AW, Kanzler S: Liver fibrosis induced by hepatic overexpression of PDGF-B in transgenic mice. *J. Hepatol.* 2006, 45:419-428.

[39] Borkham-Kamphorst E, van Roeyen CR, Ostendorf T, Floege J, Gressner AM, Weiskirchen R: Pro-fibrogenic potential of PDGF-D in liver fibrosis. *J. Hepatol.* 2007, 46:1064-1074.

[40] Friedman SL: Mechanisms of hepatic fibrogenesis. *Gastroenterology* 2008, 134:1655-1669.

[41] Bagnyukova TV, Tryndyak VP, Muskhelishvili L, Ross SA, Beland FA, Pogribny IP: Epigenetic downregulation of the suppressor of cytokine signaling 1 (Socs1) gene is associated with the STAT3 activation and development of hepatocellular carcinoma induced by methyl-deficiency in rats. *Cell Cycle* 2008, 7:3202-3210.

[42] Szabo E, Paska C, Kaposi Novak P, Schaff Z, Kiss A: Similarities and differences in hepatitis B and C virus induced hepatocarcinogenesis. *Pathol. Oncol. Res.* 2004, 10:5-11.

[43] Ikeda K, Saitoh S, Suzuki Y, Kobayashi M, Tsubota A, Koida I, Arase Y, Fukuda M, Chayama K, Murashima N, Kumada H: Disease progression and hepatocellular carcinogenesis in patients with chronic viral hepatitis: a prospective observation of 2215 patients. *J. Hepatol.* 1998, 28:930-938.

[44] Yoshikawa H, Matsubara K, Qian GS, Jackson P, Groopman JD, Manning JE, Harris CC, Herman JG: SOCS-1, a negative regulator of the JAK/STAT pathway, is silenced by methylation in human hepatocellular carcinoma and shows growth-suppression activity. *Nat. Genet.* 2001, 28:29-35.

[45] Jones PA, Baylin SB: The fundamental role of epigenetic events in cancer. *Nat. Rev. Genet.* 2002, 3:415-428.

[46] Robertson KD: DNA methylation and chromatin—unraveling the tangled web. *Oncogene* 2002, 21:5361-5379.

[47] Dhasarathy A, Wade PA: The MBD protein family—reading an epigenetic mark? *Mutat. Res.* 2008, 647:39-43.

[48] Chu PY, Yeh CM, Hsu NC, Chang YS, Chang JG, Yeh KT: Epigenetic alteration of the SOCS1 gene in hepatocellular carcinoma. *Swiss Med. Wkly.* 2010, 140:w13065.

[49] Yoshida T, Ogata H, Kamio M, Joo A, Shiraishi H, Tokunaga Y, Sata M, Nagai H, Yoshimura A: SOCS1 is a suppressor of liver fibrosis and hepatitis-induced carcinogenesis. *J. Exp. Med.* 2004, 199:1701-1707.

[50] Kaneto H, Sasaki S, Yamamoto H, Itoh F, Toyota M, Suzuki H, Ozeki I, Iwata N, Ohmura T, Satoh T, et al: Detection of hypermethylation of the p16(INK4A) gene promoter in chronic hepatitis and cirrhosis associated with hepatitis B or C virus. *Gut.* 2001, 48:372-377.

[51] Lee YH, Oh BK, Yoo JE, Yoon SM, Choi J, Kim KS, Park YN: Chromosomal instability, telomere shortening, and inactivation of

p21(WAF1/CIP1) in dysplastic nodules of hepatitis B virus-associated multistep hepatocarcinogenesis. *Mod. Pathol.* 2009, 22:1121-1131.

[52] Lee S, Lee HJ, Kim JH, Lee HS, Jang JJ, Kang GH: Aberrant CpG island hypermethylation along multistep hepatocarcinogenesis. *Am. J. Pathol* .2003, 163:1371-1378.

[53] Yang B, Guo M, Herman JG, Clark DP: Aberrant promoter methylation profiles of tumor suppressor genes in hepatocellular carcinoma. *Am. J. Pathol.* 2003, 163:1101-1107.

[54] Nishida N, Nagasaka T, Nishimura T, Ikai I, Boland CR, Goel A: Aberrant methylation of multiple tumor suppressor genes in aging liver, chronic hepatitis, and hepatocellular carcinoma. *Hepatology* 2008, 47:908-918.

[55] Oh BK, Kim H, Park HJ, Shim YH, Choi J, Park C, Park YN: DNA methyltransferase expression and DNA methylation in human hepatocellular carcinoma and their clinicopathological correlation. *Int. J. Mol. Med.* 2007, 20:65-73.

[56] Calvisi DF, Ladu S, Gorden A, Farina M, Lee JS, Conner EA, Schroeder I, Factor VM, Thorgeirsson SS: Mechanistic and prognostic significance of aberrant methylation in the molecular pathogenesis of human hepatocellular carcinoma. *J. Clin. Invest.* 2007, 117:2713-2722.

[57] Um TH, Kim H, Oh BK, Kim MS, Kim KS, Jung G, Park YN: Aberrant CpG island hypermethylation in dysplastic nodules and early HCC of hepatitis B virus-related human multistep hepatocarcinogenesis. *J. Hepatol.* 2011, 54:939-947.

In: Hepatitis C Virus
Editors: A. P. Gonzales et al.

ISBN 978-1-61942-674-0
© 2012 Nova Science Publishers, Inc.

Chapter V

Asymptomatic Low-Level Hepatitis C Virus Persistence

***Tram N. Q. Pham and Tomasz I. Michalak**[*]*
Molecular Virology and Hepatology Research Group, Division of
BioMedical Sciences, Faculty of Medicine, Health Sciences Centre,
Memorial University, St. John's, Canada

ABSTRACT

The existence of low-level hepatitis C virus (HCV) infection, termed
as occult HCV infection (OCI) has been uncovered in this laboratory by
applying assays with enhanced sensitivity and by testing patients'
samples acquired from different compartments where the virus naturally
occurs. Subsequent works conducted by us and others identified
virological and immunological characteristics of OCI, and pointed out to
potential pathological outcomes of this form of HCV infection. Occult
HCV infection can persist in the presence of antibodies against HCV
(anti-HCV) and normal liver enzymes for years after spontaneous or
interferon alpha-ribavirin (IFN/RBV) therapy-induced resolution of
hepatitis C. In addition to this residual or secondary occult infection, a
low-level HCV infection of unknown etiology in individuals negative for

---

[*] Contact information of corresponding author: Tomasz I. Michalak, MD, PhD. Molecular
Virology and Hepatology Research Group. Faculty of Medicine, Health Sciences Centre,
Memorial University, St. John's, NL, Canada A1B 3V6. Phone: (709) 777 7301 (office) or
(709) 777 7214 (lab); Fax: (709) 777 8279; Email: timich@mun.ca

anti-HCV antibodies with moderately elevated liver function enzymes has been described. This review will highlight works which led to the identification of OCI, outline known properties of the infection, present principles of OCI identification and factors influencing its detection, and summarize our current understanding of the documented and expected pathological consequences of OCI.

INTRODUCTION

Hepatitis C virus (HCV) is a human blood-borne pathogen responsible for over 170 million clinically identifiable chronic infections world-wide. However, the majority of people infected with this virus develop an asymptomatic infection where potential long-term pathological outcomes are essentially not recognized. It is generally accepted that 35% of individuals with a symptomatic acute infection spontaneously resolve hepatitis, whereas the rest become active carriers of the virus and develop chronic hepatitis C (CHC). However, up to 75% of patients with CHC may remain undiagnosed. Prolonged hepatitis C can lead to various forms of chronic liver disease, including fibrosis, cirrhosis, and hepatocellular carcinoma (HCC) [1]. While there are no prophylactic or therapeutic vaccines available for HCV, the current anti-HCV therapy is believed to slow down the progression of disease and alleviate the majority of associated clinical symptoms. Unfortunately, a vast majority of patients with CHC (up to 85%) do not receive treatment. At present, the standard antiviral treatment for patients with CHC is a combination of pegylated alpha-interferon (IFN) and ribavirin (RBV) normally administered for 24 or 48 weeks depending on the virus genotype. For example, patients infected with genotypes 1, 4 and 6 are usually treated for 48 weeks, whereas those carrying the other genotypes typically receive a 24-week treatment. It should be indicated that although this standard therapy can be successful in as much as 85% of patients infected with genotype 2 or 3, it is only effective in about 50% for patients with genotype 1 [2]. Nevertheless, very recent data demonstrate that supplementing the current IFN/RBV therapy with the newly approved protease inhibitors Telaprevir (Vertex Pharmaceuticals) or Boceprevir (Merck) significantly improve rates of sustained virological response (SVR) in treatment-experienced genotype 1 patients by as much as 4-fold [3,4].

Belonging to the *Flaviviridae* family of positive single-stranded RNA viruses, HCV is highly heterogeneous with many subtypes derived from each of the six major genotypes. The HCV genome of about 9600-base pair in length encodes for structural proteins (envelope and capsid) comprising viral particles, and a number of nonstructural proteins (NS) important for viral replication. The virus propagates by making a complementary RNA negative strand, which identification is indicative of actually progressing virus replication. Although hepatocytes are considered to be the main targets of HCV infection and the source of the majority of clinical manifestations, a number of well documented studies uncovered that the virus can also invade and replicate in extra-hepatic locations, including the lymphatic system [5]. It is perhaps the latter that may explain the over-representation of chronic HCV infection in patients with lymphoproliferative disorders, such as mixed cryoglobulinemia and non-Hodgkin's lymphoma [6,7].

HCV INFECTION OF THE LYMPHATIC SYSTEM

The notion of HCV targeting immune cells is an area of lesser recognition and much less extensively investigated. Nevertheless, those studies which examined the concept of HCV lymphotropism have revealed many unexpected and otherwise unrecognized intrinsic propensities of HCV. First, primary T cells and monocytes/macrophages, as well as cells from certain T and B cell lines, can support authentic HCV replication, as evidenced by the detection of HCV replicative intermediates, nonstructural proteins, lymphoid cell unique genome sequences and by secretion of virions [8-11]. Second, similar observations were also made in the primary immune cell subtypes derived from patients with clinically evident hepatitis C [12-15]. Moreover, the fact that culture supernatant from the ex vivo propagated lymphoid cells of some of these patients contained HCV virions capable of inducing *de novo* infection in cultured primary T cells [8,9] lend further support to the notion of HCV lymphotropism. Since this type of infection results in the appearance of HCV RNA negative (replicative) strand and intracytoplasmic viral proteins, the emergence of immune cell-specific viral variants, the release of infectious HCV-like virus particles, and the susceptibility of the virus residing in immune cells to antivirals strongly argue for HCV productively replicating in this extrahepatic compartment [8,10]. Nonetheless, it must also be indicated that the propagation of HCV in immune cells following infection with a wild-type, patient-derived virus is not nearly as robust as that found in hepatoma Huh7 cells infected with viruses generated from the HCV replicon systems and adapted to grow in culture conditions. In this context, it is noteworthy that while susceptible to plasma-derived HCV [8-11,16], immune cells do not appear to be prone to infection with the virus generated in vitro from the replicon [17]. This would suggest a potential specific modification in the viral envelope, rather than the supposed inherent inability of HCV to recognize and enter immune cells [17].

Since HCV infection of the immune system is for the most part less efficient than that of the liver, infected immune cells are unlikely to contribute significantly to the plasma viral load in patients with a symptomatic infection. However, in the course of persistent, asymptomatic, low-level infection (see below), the levels of HCV in the livers and peripheral blood lymphoid cells appear to be comparable and both these compartments may contribute to a similar degree to the pool of circulating virus. Nevertheless, by infecting immune cells, HCV likely evades immune recognition and creates a reservoir for its long-term persistence, as many viruses capable of establishing persistent infection do [18,19].

ASYMPTOMATIC LOW-LEVEL HCV PERSISTENCE

Occult HCV Infection Following Clinical Resolution of Hepatitis C

The concept of low-level HCV persistence after clinical resolution of hepatitis C, termed occult HCV infection (OCI), was first reported in 2004 following a study of 16 individuals with either spontaneous recovery or after SVR due to antiviral therapy [20]. SVR was defined at the time as HCV RNA negativity in serum by standard clinical assays for at least 6 months beyond cessation of IFN or IFN/RBV therapy. This finding of residual HCV RNA in plasma and peripheral blood mononuclear cells (PBMC) of patients convalescent from hepatitis C was highly unexpected as the widely accepted opinion had been at that time that patients with SVR would have been cured of HCV infection. In this report, the residual HCV RNA was detected by a superiorly sensitive reverse transcription (RT)-polymerase chain reaction (PCR) research assays in serum and/or PBMC of all patients investigated. HCV RNA replicative strand was identified in the majority (75%) of PBMC found reactive for HCV RNA positive strand. It appeared that the virus detection assays played a major role in the identification of minute quantities of virus genome that would have otherwise been undetectable by the standard clinical tests utilized at the time. In general terms, this RT-PCR-based research assay successively involved two rounds of PCR amplification (direct and nested) of cDNA transcribed from target samples (*i.e.,* RNA extracted from serum, PBMC or liver tissues) and nucleic acid hybridization (NAH) of amplified products using a radiolabeled HCV-specific fragment as a probe. The second step was aimed at augmenting the level of detection while simultaneously confirming the specificity of amplified species, to give the assay an overall sensitivity of $\leq$ 10 virus genome copies or virus genome equivalents (vge)/mL ($\leq$ 3 IU/mL) or $\leq$ 5 vge/µg total RNA ($\leq$ 1.5 IU/µg).

Subsequent to these initial findings, other studies also documented, using similar detection approaches, the presence of small amounts of HCV RNA in plasma or serum, PBMC and/or hepatic tissue for up to 10 years after clinical resolution of hepatitis C [21- 25]. The prevalence of OCI in individuals with SVR achieved following IFN/RBV treatment varied amongst the different studies and, depending on the number of samples per patient tested, the range of compartments investigated (*i.e.,* plasma/serum, PBMC and/or liver tissue), template preparation, sensitivity of the assays applied and how the definition of OCI was being used, the overall rate ranged between 10-100% [25]. Interestingly, although liver histology was generally and significantly improved after achieving SVR, the detectable HCV RNA in liver biopsy specimens coincided in many individuals with histological evidence of minimal to moderately active disease, including lymphocytic infiltrations, necroses of small groups or singular hepatocytes and a variable degree of fibrosis [22,23].

Certain characteristics are uniquely associated with OCI. First, HCV RNA levels are generally low, in the range of typically not higher than 200 vge/mL plasma or serum and between 10 and 100 vge/µg total RNA for circulating immune cells or liver tissue. Nevertheless, HCV genomes detected in the latter two compartments coincide, in many instances, with the simultaneous presence of the HCV RNA negative strand, implying ongoing HCV replication [20-22]. Second, *ex vivo* stimulation of peripheral immune cells, such as T cells, B cells and monocytes, with mitogens activating cell proliferation enhanced virus expression, significantly improving virus detection [20,27]. Although not necessarily unique to OCI, HCV genomes may be found predominantly in particular immune cell subsets, *e.g.,* T cells and/or B cells and/or monocytes, and that HCV occurring in these subtypes can be genetically different from the virus present in plasma [14,28,29]. Third, careful analysis of cytokine expression profiles in PBMC revealed a unique pattern of gene expression in patients with OCI compared to those with CHC or healthy individuals [25,30]. This would lend support to the notion that OCI after clinical resolution of disease is not a silent or immunologically inconsequential event.

Occult HCV Infection with Undefined Etiology

In parallel with the identification of residual/secondary HCV persistence in individuals with clinical resolution of hepatitis C, another form of low-level HCV infection was reported [31]. This form of OCI we have proposed to call cryptogenic occult HCV infection [32]. The hall-mark differences between the two types of low-level HCV infections are the level of liver function tests and reactivity of anti-HCV antibodies. Thus, in the secondary (residual) HCV infection, the patients generally have normal liver enzymes and are anti-HCV positive, whereas those with cryptogenic OCI have persistently elevated liver function tests despite a null history of hepatitis and are anti-HCV negative. In the report by Castilo *et al.* [31], HCV RNA was identifiable in liver biopsy specimens of nearly 60 individuals and in PBMC of 40 individuals from 100 patients investigated. Importantly, in the vast majority of these cases (>80%), the presence of the HCV RNA genomic (positive) strand was accompanied by that of the viral RNA replicative (negative) strand, indicating the existence of active HCV replication. As in the case with secondary OCI, the identification of cryptogenic HCV infection was made possible through the use of a highly sensitive RT-PCR-based research assay capable of detecting minute amounts of viral genome (sensitivity, 10 IU/mL) [31]. Among the most recent studies on this subject, HCV RNA was reportedly detected in about 10% of single PBMC samples obtained from 69 anti-HCV antibody-negative patients with an etiologically undefined chronic liver disease [24].

OCCULT HCV INFECTION IS NOT UNIVERSALLY DETECTED: BRIDGING THE GAPS

At this point, the existence of occult HCV infection, either secondary or cryptogenic, remains controversial. This is essentially because some studies have reported the persistent negativity, or lack-there-of, of HCV RNA in the two respective patient groups mentioned above [33,34]. In regard to secondary OCI persisting after clinical resolution of CHC due to the employed IFN/RBV treatment, the reports by George *et al.* [33] and Maylin *et al.* [34] argued that HCV RNA was not detectable in serum [33,34] or unfractionated PBMC [33] from the vast majority (>99%) of individuals who achieved SVR. Similarly, studies reported by Halfon *et al.*, [35] Nicot *et al.* [36] and Coppola *et al.* [37] submitted that HCV RNA was not present in plasma or serum, PBMC or liver tissues in patients with elevated liver enzymes of undefined etiology. Considering the expected pathogenic and epidemiological significance of OCI and its potential effect on patient care, and the apparently equally compelling findings of both for and against the existence of low-level HCV infection, one could not help but ask the questions what are the reasons behind this inconsistency and how eventually these gaps could be bridged?

First, as already stated above, the levels of HCV RNA in OCI are generally very low. Therefore, subtle differences in how patients' material is processed, preserved and analyzed, as well as variations in the sensitivity of assays used in different laboratories may cumulatively influence the efficiency with which the virus is detected. In this context, the quality and yield of recovered RNA from the patients' samples (*e.g.*, plasma, circulating cells or liver tissue) are of principal significance since their inappropriate handlings or delays in processing would lead to a loss of HCV RNA [25]. The use of commercially available RNA extraction kits does not always guarantee optimal recovery when these factors are overlooked. Second, since HCV loads tend to fluctuate in the course of OCI, testing serially collected samples and using non-standard quantities of plasma/serum, PBMC or liver biopsy for RNA extraction may be necessary to properly identify or credibly exclude virus presence [25,26,38]. Third, mitogen stimulation has been shown to upregulate HCV RNA synthesis in infected circulating immune cells by enhancing virus replication [20,27]. This means that testing of untreated PBMC may significantly underestimate the frequency of OCI occurrence [14,25]. Fourth, since HCV occurs in different immune cell subsets in different patients [14,28,29], examining HCV RNA in the unfractionated PBMC population alone may lead to falsely negative results.

In a nut shell, the elements mentioned above plus the variable sensitivities of detection assays used in different laboratories and, to some degree, the ill-defined exactness of an international unit (IU) (*i.e.*, 2 to 7 vge per 1 IU) [39] are behind the contradictory data on identification of both secondary and cryptogenic occult HCV infections.

CLINICAL RELEVANCE OF OCCULT HCV INFECTION: TO BE OR NOT TO BE?

It has been well recognized that successful antiviral therapy significantly improves clinical outcomes of CHC [40]. In the majority of patients who achieved SVR, post-treatment liver biopsies revealed an improvement in inflammation and fibrosis scores. Nevertheless, the observation is not universal as at least a subset of individuals does exhibit histological evidence of persistent hepatic inflammation characterized by periportal and intralobular minimal to moderate lymphocytic infiltrations, limited hepatocyte necrosis, and variable degree of fibrosis [21-23,26]. In the context of secondary OCI, the studies showed that histological activity of the protracted liver disease was more pronounced in patients with detectable hepatic HCV RNA, although the levels of HCV RNA did not correlate with the extent of fibrosis [21,22]. Interestingly, similar findings have also been reported for patients with cryptogenic OCI [31,41]. In fact, histological examinations of liver biopsies from individuals with an etiologically undefined liver disease recorded a higher frequency (~30%) of patients with necroinflammatory lesions, or chronic hypertransaminasaemia, having concurrent low-level HCV or HBV infection [41]. In similar cohorts, patients with detectable HCV RNA in the liver were more likely to demonstrate inflammatory lesions than those without (35% versus 14%, respectively) [31]. The continuing presence of hepatic inflammatory changes accompanied by lymphocytic infiltrations in some patients with OCI likely indicates an engagement of the cellular antiviral immune responses. Indeed, anti-HCV- positive individuals displaying normal serum levels of alanine aminotransferase (ALT; <40 IU/L) and tested HCV RNA nonreactive by standard clinical assays frequently exhibited hepatic fibrosis with CD4+ and CD8+ T cell rich inflammatory infiltrates [42]. Considering the apparent link between OCI and persistent subclinical hepatic alterations, what remained not addressed in this study was whether applying more sensitive HCV detection techniques would reveal underlying occult HCV infection in these patients.

It is currently unclear whether OCI may contribute to reactivation of hepatitis C in situations where the immune system is compromised naturally or by therapeutic intervention. However, there are data linking relapse of HCV infection after SVR or following spontaneous resolution to immune suppression, suggesting partial restoration of antiviral immunity and incomplete eradication of HCV [43-47]. There are clinical and molecular data indicating that HCC may develop in patients following therapy-induced resolution of CHC. For example, studies of large groups of patients with SVR have recorded HCC development of 2% to 3.5% [48-51], a comparable prevalence to what has been estimated for cirrhotic CHC patients [52]. While it is likely that chronic liver injury induced by HCV infection can initiate the oncogenic process, the contribution of low-level HCV replication and the potential ensuing liver injury to the carcinogenic transformation have not been investigated.

The need of antiviral treatment of patients with OCI has not been established, despite evidence of potential benefit [53,54]. In the case of cryptogenic OCI, it has been reported that treatment of 10 such patients with IFN/RBV for 6 months led to normalization of serum ALT and transient clearance of HCV RNA from PBMC for 8 [54]. Interestingly, post-treatment liver biopsies revealed significantly reduced expression of intrahepatic HCV RNA in 5 individuals, and improvement in necroinflammation and fibrosis scores in 3. Overall, the issue of whether to treat individuals with OCI remains currently unsolved.

CONCLUSION

The occurrence of OCI following resolution of clinically evident hepatitis C appears to be a common consequence and an unwavering element of the natural history of HCV infection. On the other hand, the existence of cryptogenic OCI may be a consequence of asymptomatic exposure to the virus. Certainly, further work is required to fully recognize the nature, as well as pathogenic and epidemiological consequences of low-level HCV infection so that a clear understanding of whether there is or not a need for therapy could be established.

REFERENCES

[1] Alberti A, Chemello L, Benvegnu L. Natural History Of Hepatitis C. *J. Hepatol.* 1999; 31:17 24.

[2] Fried MW, Shiffman ML, Reddy KR, Smith C, Marinos G, Gonçales FL Jr, et al. Peginterferon Alfa-2a Plus Ribavirin For Chronic Hepatitis C Infection. *N. Engl. J. Med.* 2002; 347:975-982.

[3] Zeuzem S, Andreone P, Pol S, Lawitz E, Diago M, Roberts S, et al. Telaprevir For Retreatment Of Hcv Infection. *N. Engl. J. Med.* 2011; 364:2417-2428.

[4] Fried MW. The Role Of Triple Therapy In Hcv Genotype 1-Experienced Patients. *Liver Int.* 2011; 31:58-61

[5] Blackard JT, Kemmer N, Sherman KE. Extrahepatic Replication Of Hcv: Insights Into Clinical Manifestations And Biological Consequences. *Hepatology* 2006; 44:15-22.

[6] Zignego AL, Ferri C, Giannini C, La Civita L, Careccia G, Longombardo G, et al. Hepatitis C Virus Infection In Mixed Cryoglobulinemia And B Cell Non-Hodgkin's Lymphoma: Evidence For A Pathogenic Role. *Arch. Virol.* 1997; 142:545-555.

[7] Ferri C, Monti M, La Civita L, Longombardo G, Greco F, Pasero G, et al. Infection Of Peripheral Blood Mononuclear Cells By Hepatitis C Virus In Mixed Cryoglobulinemia. *Blood* 1993; 82:3701-3704.

[8] MacParland SA, Pham TNQ, Gujar SA, Michalak TI. De Novo Infection And Propagation Of Wild-Type Hepatitis C Virus In Human T Lymphocytes In Vitro. *J. Gen. Virol.* 2006;87:3577-3586.

[9] Kondo Y, Sung VM, Machida K, Liu M, Lai MM. Hepatitis C Virus Infects T Cells And Affects Interferon-Gamma Signaling In T Cell Lines. *Virology* 2007; 361:161-173.

[10] Morsica G, Tambussi G, Sitia G, Novati R, Lazzarin A, Lopalco L, Mukenge S. Replication Of Hepatitis C Virus In B Lymphocytes (Cd19+). *Blood* 1999; 94:1138-1139.

[11] Laskus T, Radkowski M, Jablonska J, Kibler K, Wilkinson J, Adair D, Rakela J. Human Immunodeficiency Virus Facilitates Infection/Replication Of Hepatitis C Virus In Native Human Macrophages. *Blood* 2004; 103: 3854-3859.

[12] Lerat H, Rumin S, Habersetzer F, et al. In Vivo Tropism Of Hepatitis C Virus Genomic Sequences In Hematopoietic Cells: Influence Of Viral Load, Viral Genotype, And Cell Phenotype. *Blood* 1998; 91:3841-3849.

[13] Pal S, Sullivan DG, Kim S, et al. Productive Replication Of Hepatitis C Virus In Perihepatic Lymph Nodes In Vivo: Implications Of Hcv Lymphotropism. *Gastroenterology* 2006; 130:1107-1116.

[14] Pham TNQ, King D, MacParland SA, Mcgrath JS, Reddy SB, Bursey FR, Michalak TI. Hepatitis C Virus Replicates In The Same Immune Cell Subsets In Chronic Hepatitis C And Occult Infection. *Gastroenterology* 2008; 134:812-822.

[15]   Zignego AL, Macchia D, Monti M, Thiers V, Mazzetti M, Foschi M, et al. Infection Of Peripheral Mononuclear Blood Cells By Hepatitis C Virus. *J. Hepatol.* 1992; 15:382-386.

[16]   MacParland SA, Pham TNQ, Guy CS, Michalak TI. Hepatitis V Virus Persisting After Clinically Apparent Sustained Virological Response To Antiviral Therapy Retains Infectivity In Vitro. *Hepatology* 2009; 49:1431-1441.

[17]   Marukian S, Jones CT, Andrus L, Evans MJ, Ritola KD, Charles ED, et al. Cell Culture-Produced Hepatitis C Virus Does Not Infect Peripheral Blood Mononuclear Cells. *Hepatology* 2008; 48:1843-1850.

[18]   Oldstone MB. Virus-Lymphoid Cell Interactions. *Proc. Natl. Acad. Sci. USA.* 1996; 93:12756-12758.

[19]   Grosjean I, Caux C, Bella I, Berger I, Wild F, Banchereau J, Kaiserlian D. *Measles Virus Infects Human Dendritic Cells And Blocks Their Allostimulatory Property For CD4$^+$ T Cells. J. Exp. Med. 1997; 186: 801-812.*

[20]   Pham TNQ, MacParland SA, Mulrooney PM, Cooksley H, Naoumov NV, Michalak TI. Hepatitis C Virus Persistence after Spontaneous Or Treatment-Induced Resolution Of Hepatitis C. *J. Virol.* 2004; 78: 5867-5874.

[21]   Ciancio A, Smedile A, Giordanino C, Colletta C, Croce G, Pozzi M, et al. Long Term Follow-Up Of Previous Hepatitis C Virus Positive Nonresponders To Interferon Monotherapy Successfully Retreated With Combination Therapy: Are They Really Cured? *Am. J. Gastroenterol.* 2006; 101:1811-1816.

[22]   Castillo I, Rodriguez-Inigo E, Lopez-Alcorocho JM, Pardo M, Bartolome J, Carreno V. Hepatitis C Virus Replicates In The Liver Of Patients Who Have A Sustained Response To Antiviral Treatment. *Clin. Infect. Dis.* 2006; 43:1277-1283.

[23]   Radkowski M, Gallegos-Orozco JF, Jablonska J, Colby TV, Walewska-Zielecka B, Kubicka J, et al. Persistence Of Hepatitis C Virus In Patients Successfully Treated For Chronic Hepatitis C. *Hepatology* 2005;41:106-114.

[24]   Zaghloul H, El Sherbiny W. Detection Of Occult Hepatitis C And Hepatitis B Virus Infections From Peripheral Blood Mononuclear Cells. *Immunol. Invest.* 2010; 39:284-291.

[25]   Pham TNQ, Coffin CS, Michalak TI. Occult Hepatitis C Virus Infection: What Does It Mean? *Liver Int.* 2010; 30:502-511.

[26] Pham TNQ, Coffin CS, Churchill ND, Urbanski SJ, Lee SS, Michalak TI. Hepatitis C Virus Persistence After Sustained Virological Response To Antiviral Therapy In Patients With Or Without Past Exposure To Hepatitis B Virus. *J. Viral. Hepat.* 2011 (Published Online March 1, 2011).

[27] Pham TNQ, MacParland SA, Coffin CS, Lee SS, Bursey FR, Michalak, TI. Mitogen-Induced Upregulation Of Hepatitis C Virus Expression In Human Lymphoid Cells. *J. Gen. Virol.* 2005; 86:657-666.

[28] Di Liberto G, Roque-Afonso AM, Kara R, Ducoulombier D, Fallot G, Samuel D, Feray C. Clinical And Therapeutic Implications Of Hepatitis C Virus Compartmentalization. *Gastroenterology* 2006; 131:76-84.

[29] Ducoulombier D, Roque-Afonso AM, Di Liberto G, Penin F, Kara R, Richard Y, Dussaix E, et al. Frequent Compartmentalization Of Hepatitis C Virus Variants In Circulating B Cells And Monocytes. *Hepatology* 2004; 39:817-825.

[30] Pham TNQ, Mercer SE, Michalak TI. Chronic Hepatitis C And Persistent Occult Hepatitis C Virus Infection Are Characterized By Distinct Immune Cell Cytokine Expression Profiles. *J. Viral. Hepat.* 2009; 16:547-556.

[31] Castillo I, Pardo M, Bartolome J, Ortiz-Movilla N, Rodríguez-Iñigo E, De Lucas S, et al. Occult Hepatitis C Virus Infection In Patients In Whom The Etiology Of Persistently Abnormal Results Of Liver-Function Tests Is Unknown. *J. Infect. Dis.* 2004; 189:7-14.

[32] Michalak TI, Pham TNQ. Anti-Hcv Core Antibody: A Potential New Marker Of Occult And Otherwise Serologically Silent HCV Infection. *J. Hepatol.* 2009; 50: 244-246.

[33] George SL, Bacon BR, Brunt EM, Mihindukulasuriya KL, Hoffmann J, Di Bisceglie AM. Clinical, Virologic, Histologic, And Biochemical Outcomes After Successful HCV Therapy: A 5-Year Follow-Up Of 150 Patients. *Hepatology* 2009;49:729-738.

[34] Maylin S, Martinot-Peignoux M, Ripault MP, Moucari R, Cardoso AC, Boyer N, et al. Sustained Virological Response Is Associated With Clearance Of Hepatitis C Virus RNA And A Decrease In Hepatitis C Virus Antibody. *Liver Int.* 2009;29:511-517.

[35] Halfon P, Bourliere M, Ouzan D, Sène D, Saadoun D, Khiri H, et al. Occult Hepatitis C Virus Infection Revisited With Ultrasensitive Real-Time PCR Assay. *J. Clin. Microbiol.* 2008; 46:2106-2108.

[36] Nicot F, Kamar N, Mariame B, Rostaing L, Pasquier C, Izopet J. No Evidence of Occult Hepatitis C Virus (HCV) Infection In Serum Of

HCV Antibody-Positive HCV RNA-Negative Kidney-Transplant Patients. *Transpl. Int.* 2010;23:594-601.

[37]   Coppola N, Pisaturo M, Guastafierro S, Tonziello G, Sica A, Sagnelli C, Ferrara MG, et al. Absence Of Occult HCV Infection In Patients Under Immunosupressive Therapy For Oncohematological Diseases. *Hepatology* 2011; 54:1487-1489.

[38]   Castillo I, Bartolome J, Quiroga JA, Barril G, Carreno V. Presence Of HCV-RNA After Ultracentrifugation Of Serum Samples During The Follow-Up Of Chronic Hepatitis C Patients With A Sustained Virological Response May Predict Reactivation Of Hepatitis C Virus Infection. *Aliment. Pharmacol. Ther.* 2009; 30:477-486.

[39]   Germer JJ, Zein NN. Advances In The Molecular Diagnosis Of Hepatitis C And Their Clinical Implications. *Mayo Clin. Proc.* 2001; 76:911-920.

[40]   Formann E, Steindl-Munda P, Hofer H, Jessner W, Bergholz U, Gurguta C, Ferenci P. Long-Term Follow-Up Of Chronic Hepatitis C Patients With Sustained Virological Response To Various Forms Of Interferon-Based Anti-Viral Therapy. *Aliment. Pharmacol. Ther.* 2006; 23: 507-511.

[41]   Berasain C, Betes M, Panizo A, Ruiz J, Herrero JI, Civeira MP, Prieto J. Pathological And Virological Findings In Patients With Persistent Hypertransaminasaemia Of Unknown Aetiology. *Gut* 2000; 47:429-435.

[42]   Hoare M, Gelson WT, Rushbrook SM, Curran MD, Woodall T, Coleman N, Davies SE. Histological Changes In HCV Antibody-Positive, HCV RNA-Negative Subjects Suggest Persistent Virus Infection. *Hepatology* 2008; 48:1737-1745.

[43]   Charlton M, Seaberg E, Wiesner R, Everhart J, Zetterman R, Lake J, et al. Predictors Of Patient And Graft Survival Following Liver Transplantation Fror Hepatitis C. *Hepatology* 1998; 28:823-830.

[44]   Lee WM, Polson JE, Carney DS, Sahin B, Gale M, Jr. Reemergence Of Hepatitis C Virus After 8.5 Years In A Patient With Hypogammaglobulinemia. Evidence For An Occult Viral Reservoir. *J. Infect. Dis.* 2005; 192:1088-1092.

[45]   Lin A, Thadareddy A, Goldstein MJ, Lake-Bakaar G. Immune Suppression Leading To Hepatitis C Virus Re-Emergence After Sustained Virological Response. *J. Med. Virol.* 2008; 80:1720-1722.

[46]   Nudo CG, Cortes RA, Weppler D, Schiff ER, Tzakis AG, Regev A. Effect Of Pretransplant Hepatitis C Virus RNA Status On Posttransplant Outcome. *Transplant Proc.* 2008; 40:1449-1455.

[47] Thomopoulos K, Giannakoulas NC, Tsamandas AC, Mimidis K, Fragopanagou E, Pallasopoulou M, Lampropoulou-Karatza CH. Recurrence Of HCV Infection In A Sustained Responder After Chemotherapy For Non-Hodgkin's Lymphoma: Successful Retreatment. *Am. J. Med. Sci.* 2008; 336:73-76.

[48] Kobayashi S, Takeda T, Enomoto M, Tamori A, Kawada N, Habu D, et al. Development Of Hepatocellular Carcinoma In Patients With Chronic Hepatitis C Who Had A Sustained Virological Response To Interferon Therapy: A Multicenter, Retrospective Cohort Study Of 1124 Patients. *Liver Int.* 2007; 27:186-191.

[49] Makiyama A, Itoh Y, Kasahara A, Tamori A, Kawada N, Habu D, et al. Characteristics Of Patients With Chronic Hepatitis C Who Develop Hepatocellular Carcinoma After A Sustained Response To Interferon Therapy. *Cancer* 2004; 101:1616-1622.

[50] Veldt BJ, Saracco G, Boyer N, Cammà C, Bellobuono A, Hopf U, et al. Long Term Clinical Outcome Of Chronic Hepatitis C Patients With Sustained Virological Response To Interferon Monotherapy. *Gut* 2004; 53:1504-1508.

[51] Veldt BJ, Heathcote EJ, Wedemeyer H, Reichen J, Hofmann WP, Zeuzem S, et al. Sustained Virologic Response And Clinical Outcomes In Patients With Chronic Hepatitis C And Advanced Fibrosis. *Ann. Intern. Med.* 2007; 147:677-684.

[52] Freeman AJ, Dore GJ, Law MG, Thorpe M, Von Overbeck J, Lloyd AR, et al. Estimating Progression To Cirrhosis In Chronic Hepatitis C Virus Infection. *Hepatology* 2001; 34:809-816.

[53] Casato M, Lilli D, Donato G, Granata M, Conti V, Del Giudice G, et al. Occult Hepatitis C Virus Infection In Type Ii Mixed Cryoglobulinaemia. *J. Viral. Hepat.* 2003; 10:455-459.

[54] Pardo M, Castillo I, Rodriguez-Inigo E. Antiviral Therapy In Patients With Occult Hcv Infection. *Hepatology* 2005; 42:658a.

In: Hepatitis C Virus
Editors: A. P. Gonzales et al.

ISBN 978-1-61942-674-0
© 2012 Nova Science Publishers, Inc.

Chapter VI

Clinicopathological Approach of HCV Infection in Renal Transplant Recipients

Johanna Delladetsima and Stratigoula Sakellariou
1st Department of Pathology, Medical School, Athens University,
Athens, Greece

ABSTRACT

HCV infection is the leading cause of liver disease in renal transplant (RTx) recipients. Despite its high frequency, the impact of immunosuppression on the evolution of the disease remains unclear while histopathological changes have not been thoroughly investigated.

Data referring to patients' survival and hepatitis progression are still controversial. According to some reports, chronic hepatitis C (CHC) runs a rather benign course after transplantation showing a short-term survival similar to non-infected patients without significant difference in the severity of liver disease between hemodialysis and transplant patients. On the contrary, other studies demonstrated an adverse clinical outcome, especially after long-term follow-up. Although prognostic factors have not yet been precisely defined, duration of hepatitis and the severity of pre-existing liver disease seem to influence disease progression. Moreover, some data suggest that time of acquisition of HCV infection in relation to transplantation may present a prognostic parameter playing a significant role in hepatitis evolution. The majority of RTx recipients are infected with HCV while being on hemodialysis. A small number of patients acquire the infection shortly before, rarely during transplantation, and occasionally in the post-transplant period. There are indications that patients showing a milder clinical course were contaminated before transplantation and during the time period spent on hemodialysis. On the contrary, patients infected close to or after transplantation display an adverse hepatitis outcome.

Histologically, HCV infection presents as conventional acute and chronic hepatitis and rarely as fibrosing cholestatic hepatitis (FCH) and interlobular bile duct damage and loss. Acute hepatitis is generally mild. Chronic hepatitis is minimal or mild and only exceptionally of moderate severity. FCH and interlobular bile duct damage and loss occur mostly during the early and late post-transplant period, respectively. Liver cell apoptosis seems to be an important factor in liver injury closely linked to high viral load. The direct pathogenetic role of HCV is further supported by the association of both cholestatic syndromes and an adverse hepatitis evolution with high viremia levels.

Conclusively, time point of infection seems to be of major prognostic significance rendering immunosuppression as a crucial prognostic factor in the evolvement of hepatitis in patients that are infected at the time or after transplantation. The histological range includes besides conventional acute and chronic hepatitis, cholestatic diseases such as FCH and bile duct damage and loss. High viral load seems to play an important role in the pathogenesis, rendering an early reduction of the immunosuppressive therapy mandatory.

NATURAL COURSE

HCV infection is the leading cause of liver disease in renal transplant (RTx) recipients. Despite its high frequency, the impact of immunosuppression on the evolution of the disease remains obscure; data referring to patient's survival and hepatitis progression are controversial while histopathological changes have not been thoroughly investigated. There are reports of a relatively mild hepatitis course showing short-term survival similar to non-infected transplanted patients and no remarkable differences in the severity of the disease during hemodialysis and after transplantation [1-5]. Slow progression and even regression of fibrosis has been observed in the postransplantation period [6-8]. Conversely, other investigations documented an adverse clinical outcome and increased mortality especially after long term follow up [9-15].

These discrepancies may result from variations in hepatitis duration, follow-up period, severity of preexistent liver disease and kind of immunosuppressive therapy. Moreover, the time of acquisition of HCV infection in relation to transplantation has been proposed as a contributory factor in the evolution of liver disease [16-18]. In the majority of RTx recipients, HCV infection preexists, having being acquired during the time spent on hemodialysis. However, a limited number of patients run the acute phase of primary infection under immunosuppression, being infected shortly before transplantation, rarely during transplantation from HCV- positive donors or occasionally in the post-transplantation period. There are strong indications derived from a few studies and case reports that HCV infection acquired close to or after renal transplantation and under immunosuppression, is associated with an adverse clinical outcome, characterized by rapid progression of fibrosis, development of cholestatic syndromes and high mortality rate, reaching 30% in a 6 years interval [16. 17. 19- 22]. Acute hepatitis occurring peri- or post-transplantation and under the influence of immunosuppressive therapy seems to be of great prognostic significance and determines a specific high-risk group of patients. Moreover, cholestatic syndromes present major complications manifesting as fibrosing cholestatic hepatitis (FCH) in the early and as vanishing bile duct syndrome (VBDS) in the late post-transplantation period [16]. On the other hand, post- transplant low progression rate and regression of fibrosis have been reported in patients who were contaminated during hemodialysis [7. 8]. The prognostic significance of the time of contamination was demonstrated in two comparative studies which showed that acquisition of HCV infection during or after transplantation was associated with severe and rapidly progressive clinicopathological course [18] and higher mortality rate [22] compared to the evolution of the disease in patients with preexistent HCV infection.

The deleterious role of immunosuppression in the peri- and post-transplant period should be ascribed to the modulation of the acute phase of HCV infection. It is well known that the efficacy of the immune system at the time of virus acquisition is crucial in determining hepatitis outcome. The inability to mount a specific immune response results in deficient control of viral replication and of hepatocellular infection. Most probably a condition of virus tolerance is created which cannot be overturned as long as the patient is under immunosuppression. Conversely, immunosuppressive therapy does not seem to affect substantially the functional properties of the specific immune reaction generated in the immunocompetent phase of infection. Most probably, after transplantation, the immune response retains an adequate efficacy prohibiting an overwhelming virus replication.

HISTOLOGY

The complex interplay between immunosupression, virus replication and immune system results in distinct histological entities. The pathological spectrum of HCV infection in RTx recipients includes "healthy carrier" state, conventional acute and chronic hepatitis, FCH and interlobular bile duct damage and loss. The *"healthy carrier" state* refers to HCV-RNA positive patients with normal transaminase values and non-significant changes or normal liver on histological level. A frequency of 10-14% has been assessed [1. 23. 24].

Histological data concerning *acute hepatitis* is limited suggesting mild liver damage with an increased number of apoptotic hepatocytes similarly to the histology experienced from HCV infected liver grafts [16. 25-27]. *Chronic hepatitis* is minimal or mild and only exceptionally of moderate severity [23. 24. 28], while the frequency of cirrhosis ranges between 2-21% in different reports [1. 24. 29. 30]. In one study, liver biopsies performed within a mean of 4.7 years (SD 3.6 years) after transplantation showed non-significant changes in 14% and chronic hepatitis in 86% of the cases. Minimal hepatitis was diagnosed in 54% of the patients, mild in 28%, and moderate in 3%. Advanced hepatitis stage (moderate-severe) and cirrhosis were found in 12% and 3% respectively [24]. Degenerative liver cell changes and mild ductular reaction appear to be common histological features (unpublished observations), which have also been described in chronic hepatits C in liver grafts [27]. Elementary liver lesions of chronic hepatitis C such as lymphoid aggregates and lymphocytic cholangitis are less commonly encountered compared to the general population while steatosis exhibits almost the same prevalence [31-33].

Fibrosing cholestatic hepatitis presents a rare complication of HCV infection usually acquired in the early transplant period during the time of maximal immunosuppression. It is associated with high HCV viremia levels while anti-HCV antibodies may be absent. The disease leads to the development of liver failure, usually within few months [26]. It has also been described in other highly immunocompromised patients and was initially introduced in HBV infected liver grafts [25. 27]. In a series of renal transplant recipients with HCV infection, FCH was recognized in 5% of the patients [26]. A direct cytopathic effect of the virus is implicated in the pathogenesis due to uncontrolled replication and massive intracellular accumulation [25. 26. 34]. The intrahepatic immune response in HCV-related FCH is reported to be TH-2–like and the few infiltrating lymphocytes often lack HCV specificity [35]. The predominant histological features of FCH are ballooning of hepatocytes, prominent ductular reaction and perisinusoidal fibrosis, primarily limited to acinar zone 1 and progressively extending deep into the parenchyma. Acidophilic bodies, focal cell loss, bilirubinostasis and non significant portal inflammation present additional findings [26. 27. 36]. In liver transplants, cholestasis and fibrosis in association with recurrent hepatitis C were considered early signs of FCH development [37]. Regression of histological lesions of FCH in renal allograft recipients has been observed after drastic reduction of immunosuppression [26. 36].

Damage and loss of interlobular bile ducts is a rare complication of HCV infection occurring in the late post-transplant period [16. 38]. It manifests as a cholestatic syndrome appearing simultaneously or within an interval of 2–4 years after the detection of anti-HCV antibodies. The biochemical profile of cholestasis is histologically associated with lesions of the small-sized interlobular bile ducts. Early bile duct abnormalities are of mild degree and are characterized mainly by vacuolar cytoplasmic degeneration and nuclear irregularity. Late and more severe biliary lesions acquire features of bile duct vanishing syndrome including bile duct destruction and loss [38]. Coexisting findings of chronic hepatitis were found in milder lesions while chronic cholestasis predominated in more severe forms. In half of the patients (two out of four) progressive VBDS led to liver failure and death, 2 and 3 years after disease biochemical onset. In the other half, marked improvement of liver function was achieved after drastic reduction and cessation of immunosuppression [38]. The onset of the cholestatic syndrome in relation to the detection of anti-HCV antibodies, the association of disease progression with high HCV RNA levels and disease remission after withdrawal or drastic reduction of immunosuppression, speak in favour of a direct cytopathic effect of high viral load. As long as biliary cells constitute an appropriate host of HCV [39], one may assume that an unrestricted virus replication and intracellular accumulation may lead to bile duct epithelium damage, although a synergistic impact of immunosuppressive drugs cannot be excluded [40]. In immunocompetent patients HCV has been implicated as a putative cause of idiopathic adulthood ductopenia [41].

PATHOGENESIS

The pathogenesis of chronic hepatitis C in immunocompetent patients relies on specific and non-specific immune response. The combination of Th1 immune reaction through cytotoxic T lymphocytes as well as indirect nonspecific pathways are implicated for liver damage in hepatits C re-infection after liver transplantation [42-45]. High HCV RNA levels trigger an ineffective immune response leading to hepatocellular damage, while HCV overload is suggested to be involved in direct cytotoxic pathways in cholestatic complications [34]. In the setting of renal graft recipients strong indications of a direct cytopathic HCV involvement in liver injury are provided not only by the markedly elevated viremia levels in both cholestatic syndromes but also by the high viral burden in the patients group with an adverse post-transplant clinical outcome [16]. The interference of the virus in the pathogenetic process is further supported by the postulated association of apoptotic cell death with high viral load in HCV infected liver transplant recipients. A correlation of apoptosis with high viremia levels was identified irrespective of hepatitis grade, lobular activity, and CD8 T-cell count [24]. This hypothesis is further enhanced by the detection of a high apoptotic index in biopsies showing no significant changes or minimal hepatitis [24] as well as in histologically normal allografts [46. 47]. HCV is directly involved in the pathogenesis of liver cell apoptosis probably by modulating the apoptotic pathways through interaction with apoptosis mediators. In favor of this assumption are experimental data confirming that the contribution of HCV proteins in the apoptotic mechanisms is possible. In vitro studies using different cell lines have shown that actually all HCV proteins have pro and anti-apoptotic properties [48]. In particular, the multipotential core protein as a pro-apoptotic factor binds to the cytoplasmic domain of tumor necrosis factor receptor 1, lymphotoxin-β receptor and Fas [49-51], while NS3 and NS5 proteins have been related to anti-apoptotic effects [52-54]. Other experimental data suggest a direct apoptotic effect of HCV E1 and E2 proteins, the latter through a mitochondrial-related caspase pathway [55. 56].

The potential role of HCV genotype in the evolution of the disease is still unknown. The high frequency of genotype 1 in patients with both cholestatic syndromes [26. 38] suggests a possible impact in their pathogenesis, a hypothesis enhanced by similar observations deriving from FCH in liver transplants [57. 58].

Data regarding quasispecies are poor and suggest an association of slow quasispecies diversification with liver fibrosis progression in renal transplants

[28] , while in liver allografts cholestatic hepatitis C recurrence was correlated not only with high viral load but also with stable quasispecies [59. 60].

Another issue under investigation is the influence of immunosuppressive drugs on the outcome of hepatitis mainly by affecting HCV replication. Azathioprine, anti-lymphocyte globulin, anti-thymocyte globulin and OKT3 have been associated with worsening [29. 61], while antiviral effects of cyclosporine (CsA) remain controversial [61-66], probably due to a diverse virus sensitivity to CsA, related to polymorphisms of nonstructural HCV proteins NS5A and NS5B [67]. The impact of mycophenolate mofetil (MMF) therapy on viral replication and the disease itself is also obscure due to different observations regarding viremia levels after drug administration [68-70].

CONCLUSION REMARKS

Renal graft recipients with HCV infection should be monitored regularly for liver biochemistry, while follow up biopsies are mandatory especially for the group of patients infected in the peri- and posttransplant period. In the pretransplantation anti-HCV negative setting, biochemical liver dysfunction constitutes absolute indication for HCV serology testing and HCV RNA examination, as well as for liver biopsy performance. Early diagnosis of a recent HCV infection and of deterioration of liver disease is crucial for further therapeutic intervention.

REFERENCES

[1]   Dominguez-Gil B, Morales J M. Transplantation in the patient with hepatitis C. *Tranplant Int.* 2009 Dec; 22 (12): 1117-31.

[2]   Glicklich D, Thung SN, Kapoian T, Tellis V, Reinus JF. Comparison of clinical features and liver histology in hepatitis C-positive dialysis patients and renal transplant recipients. *Am J Gastroenterol 1999 Jan;* 94(1): 159-63.

[3]   Collier J, Heathcote J. Hepatitis C viral infection in the immunosuppressed patient. *Hepatology* 1998 Jan; 27 (1):2-6.

[4]   Roth D, Zucker K, Cirocco R, Burke G, Ciancio G, Esquenazi V, Swanson SJ 3rd, Miller J. A prospective study of hepatitis C virus

infection in renal allograft recipients. *Transplantation* 1996 Mar 27; 61:886-9.

[5]   Chan TM, Lok AS, Cheng IK, Chan RT. A prospective study of hepatitis C virus infection among renal transplant recipients. *Gastroenterology* 1993 Mar; 104 (3):862-8.

[6]   Roth D, Gaynor JJ, Reddy KR, Ciancio G, Sageshima J, Kupin W, Guerra G, Chen L, Burke GW 3rd. Effect of kidney transplantation on outcomes among patients with hepatitis C. *J Am Soc Nephrol.* 2011; Jun 22(6):1152-60.

[7]   Kamar N, Rostaing L, Selves J, Sandres-Saune K, Alric L, Durand D, Izopet J. Natural history of hepatitis C virus-related liver fibrosis after renal transplantation. *Am J Transplant.* 2005 Jul; 5(7):1704-12.

[8]   Alric L, Di-Martino V, Selves J, Cacoub P, Charlotte F, Reynaud D, Piette JC, Péron JM, Vinel JP, Durand D, Izopet J, Poynard T, Duffaut M, Rostaing L. Long-term impact of renal transplantation on liver fibrosis during hepatitis C virus infection. *Gastroenterology* 2002 Nov; 123(5):1494-9.

[9]   Mathurin P, Mouquet C, Poynard T, Sylla C, Benalia H, Fretz C, Thibault V, Cadranel JF, Bernard B, Opolon P, Coriat P, Bitker MO. Impact of hepatitis B and C virus on kidney transplantation outcome. *Hepatology* 1999 Jan; 29 (1): 257-63.

[10]   Fabrizi F, Martini P, Ponticelli C. Hepatitis C virus infection and renal transplantation. *Am J Kidney Dis* 2001 Nov; 38 (5): 919-34.

[11]   Pereira BJ, Wright TL, Schmid CH, Levey AS. The impact of pretransplantation hepatitis C infection on the outcome of renal transplantation. *Transplantation* 1995 Oct 27; 60 (8):799-805.

[12]   Hanafusa T, Ichikawa Y, Kishikawa H, Kyo M, Fukunishi T, Kokado Y, Okuyama A, Shinji Y, Nagano S. Retrospective study on the impact of hepatitis C virus infection on kidney transplant patients over 20 years. *Transplantation* 1998 Aug 27; 66 (4):471-6.

[13]   Fabrizi F, Martin P, Dixit V, Bunnapradist S, Dulai G. Hepatitis C virus antibody status and survival after renal transplantation: meta-analysis of observational studies. *Am J Transplant* 2005 Jun; 5 (6):1452-61.

[14]   Meyers CM, Seeff LB, Stehman-Breen CO, Hoofnagle JH. Hepatitis C and renal disease: an update. *Am J Kidney Dis* 2003 Oct; 42 (4): 631-57.

[15]   Ridruejo E, Díaz C, Michel MD, Soler Pujol G, Martínez A, Marciano S, Mandó OG, Vilches A. Short and long term outcome of kidney transplanted patients with chronic viral hepatitis B and C. *Ann Hepatol.* 2010 Jul-Sep; 9(3):271-7

[16] Delladetsima I, Psichogiou M, Sypsa V, Psimenou E, Kostakis A, Hatzakis A, Boletis JN. The course of hepatitis C virus infection in pretransplantation anti-hepatitis C virus-negative renal transplant recipients: a retrospective follow-up study. *Am J Kidney Dis* 2006 Feb; 47 (2):309-16.

[17] Ok E, Unsal A, Celik A, Zeytinoglu A, Ersoz G, Tokat Y, Erensoy S, Akarca US, Basçi A, Yüce G. Clinicopathological features of rapidly progressive hepatitis C virus infection in HCV antibody negative renal transplant recipients. *Nephrol Dial Transpl* 1998 Dec; 13 (12): 3103-7.

[18] Töz H, Nart D, Turan I, Ersöz G, Seziş M, Aşçi G, Ozkahya M, Zeytinoğlu A, Erensoy S, Ok E. The acquisition time of infection: a determinant of the severity of hepatitis C virus-related liver disease in renal transplant patients. *Clin Tranplant.* 2009 Sep-Oct; 23 (5): 723-31.

[19] Pereira BJ, Levey AS. Hepatitis C virus infection in dialysis and renal transplantation. *Kidney Int* 1997 Apr; 51 (4):981-99.

[20] Chan TM, Wu PC, Lok AS, Lai CL, Cheng IK. Clinicopathological features of hepatitis C virus antibody negative fatal chronic hepatitis C after renal transplantation. *Nephron* 1995; 71 (2) 213-7.

[21] Dussol B, Brunet P, Cantaloube JF, Schleinitz N, Biagnini P, Berland Y. Hepatitis C virus infection contracted just before kidney transplantation. *Nephron* 1995; 71 (2): 229.

[22] Breitenfeldt MK, Rasenack J, Berhold H, Olschewksi M, Schroff J, Strey C, Grotz WH. Impact of hepatitis B and C on graft loss and mortality of patients after kidney transplantation. *Clin Transplant* 2002; Apr; 16 (2):130-6.

[23] Sandrini S, Chiappini R, Setti G, Carli O, Matricardi L, Puoti M, Callea F, Favret M, Maiorca R. Hepatitis C virus infection after renal transplantation: prevalence and course of morphologic lesions. *Transplant Proc.* 1998 Aug; 30(5):2100-1.

[24] Delladetsima I, Psichogiou M, Alexandrou P, Nikolopoulos G, Revenas K, Hatzakis A, Boletis J. Apoptosis and hepatitis C virus infection in renal transplant recipients. *Am J Clin Pathol* 2008 May; 129(5): 744-8

[25] McCaughan GW, Zekry A. Pathogenesis of hepatitis C virus recurrence in the liver allograft. Liver Transpl. 2002 Oct; 8 (10 Suppl 1): S7-S13.

[26] Delladetsima KJ, Boletis NJ, Makris F, Psichogiou M, Kostakis A, Hatzakis A. Fibrosing cholestatic hepatitis in renal transplant recipients with hepatitis C virus infection. *Liver Transpl Surg.* 1999 Jul; 5 (4): 294-300.

[27] Demetris AJ. Evolution of hepatitis C virus in liver allografts. *Liver Transpl.* 2009 Nov; 15 Suppl 2:S35-41.

[28] Izopet J, Rostaing L, Sandres K, Cisterne JM, Pasquier C, Rumeau JL, Duffaut M, Durand D, Puel J. Longitudinal analysis of hepatitis C virus replication and liver fibrosis progression in renal transplant recipients. *J Infect Dis.* 2000 Mar; 181(3):852-8.

[29] Vosnides GG. Hepatitis C in renal transplantation. *Kidney Int* 1997; Sep; 52(3):843-61.

[30] Zylberberg H, Nalpas B, Carnot F, Skhiri H, Fontaine H, Legendre C, Kreis H, Bréchot C, Pol S. Severe evolution of chronic hepatitis C in renal transplantation: a case control study. *Nephrol Dial Transplant* 2002 Jan; 17(1):129-33.

[31] Perez RM, Ferreira AS, Medina-Pestana JO, Cendoroglo-Neto M, Lanzoni VP, Silva AE, Ferraz ML. Is hepatitis C more aggressive in renal transplant patients than in patients with end-stage renal disease? *J Clin Gastroenterol.* 2006 May-Jun; 40(5):444-8.

[32] Delladetsima JK, Rassidakis G, Tassopoulos NC, Papatheodoridis GV, Smyrnoff T, Vafiadis I. Histopathology of chronic hepatitis C in relation to epidemiological factors. *J Hepatol.* 1996 Jan; 24(1):27-32.

[33] Delladetsima JK, Boletis J, Makris F, Katsoulidou A, Vafiadis I, Kostakis A, Hatzakis A, Vosnides G. Histopathology of HCV infection in renal transplant patients. *J Hepatol.* 1995; 23 (Suppl 1):101.

[34] McCaughan GW, Zekry A. Mechanisms of HCV reinfection and allograft damage after liver transplantation. *J Hepatol* 2004; 40: 368-74.

[35] Zekry A, Bishop GA, Bowen DG, Gleeson MM, Guney S, Painter DM, McCaughan GW. Intrahepatic cytokine profiles associated with posttransplantation hepatitis C virus related liver injury. *Liver Transpl* 2002 Mar; 8 (3): 292-301.

[36] Xiao SY, Lu L, Wang HL. Fibrosing cholestatic hepatitis: clinicopathologic spectrum, diagnosis and pathogenesis. *Int J Clin Exp Pathol.* 2008 Jan 1; 1(5):396-402.

[37] Dixon LR, Crawford JM. Early histologic changes in fibrosing cholestatic hepatitis C. *Liver Transpl* 2007 Feb; 13 (2): 219-226.

[38] Delladetsima KJ, Makris F, Psichogiou M, Kostakis A, Hatzakis A, Boletis NJ. Cholestatic syndrome with bile duct damage and loss in renal transplant recipients with HCV infection. *Liver* 2001 Apr; 21 (2): 81-8.

[39] Loriot MA, Bronowicki JP, Lagorce D, Lakehal F, Persico T, Barba G, Mergey M, Vons C, Franco D, Belghiti J, Giacca M, Housset C,

Bréchot C. Permissiveness of human biliary epithelial cells to infection by hepatitis C virus. *Hepatology* 1999 May; 29 (5): 1587–95.

[40] Horsmans Y, Rahier J, Geubel AP. Reversible cholestasis with bile duct injury following azathioprine therapy. A case report. *Liver.* 1991 Apr; 11(2):89-93.

[41] Ludwig J. Idiopathic adulthood ductopenia: an update. *Mayo Clin Proc.* 1998 Mar; 73(3):285-91.

[42] Gane EJ. The natural history of recurrent hepatitis C and what influences this. *Liver Transpl* 2008 Oct; 14 Suppl 2: S36–S44.

[43] Ramirez S, Perez-Del-Pulgar S, Forns X. Virology and pathogenesis of hepatitis C virus recurrence. *Liver Transpl* 2008 Oct; 14 Suppl 2: S27–S35.

[44] McCaughan GW, Shackel NA, Bertolino P, Bowen DG. Molecular and cellular aspects of hepatitis C virus reinfection after liver transplantation: how the early phase impacts on outcomes. *Transplantation* 2009 Apr; 87 (8): 1105-11.

[45] Mengshol JA, Golden-Mason L, Rosen HR. Mechanisms of disease: HCV-induced liver injury. *Nat Clin Pract Gastroenterol Hepatol* 2007 Nov; 4 (11):622-34.

[46] Di Martino V, Brenot C, Samuel D, Saurini F, Paradis V, Reynés M, Bismuth H, Féray C. Influence of liver hepatitis C virus RNA and hepatitis C virus genotype on Fas-mediated apoptosis after liver transplantation for hepatitis C. *Transplantation.* 2000 Nov 15; 70 (9):1390-6.

[47] Ballardini G, De Raffele E, Groff P, Bioulac-Sage P, Grassi A, Ghetti S, Susca M, Strazzabosco M, Bellusci R, Iemmolo RM, Grazi G, Zauli D, Cavallari A, Bianchi FB. Timing of reinfection and mechanisms of hepatocellular damage in transplanted hepatitis C virus–reinfected liver. *Liver Transpl.* 2002 Jan; 8 (1):10-20.

[48] Fischer R, Baumert T, Blum HE. Hepatitis C virus infection and apoptosis. *World J Gastroenterol.* 2007 Sep 28; 13(36): 4865-72.

[49] Matsumoto M, Hsieh TY, Zhu N, et al. Hepatitis C virus core protein interacts with the cytoplasmic tail of lymphotoxin-beta receptor. *J Virol.* 1997; 71:1301-1309.

[50] Zhu N, Khoshnan A, Schneider R, Matsumoto M, Dennert G, Ware C, Lai MM. Hepatitis C virus core protein binds to the cytoplasmic domain of tumor necrosis factor (TNF) receptor 1 and enhances TNF-induced apoptosis. *J Virol.* 1998 May; 72 (5):3691-7.

[51] Hahn CS, Cho YG, Kang BS, Lester IM, Hahn YS. The HCV core protein acts as a positive regulator of Fas-mediated apoptosis in a human lymphoblastoid T cell line.*Virology.* 2000 Oct 10; 276 (1):127-37.

[52] Fujita T, Ishido S, Muramatsu S, Itoh M, Hotta H. Suppression of actinomycin D–induced apoptosis by the NS3 protein of hepatitis C virus. *Biochem Biophys Res Commun.* 1996 Dec 24; 229 (3):825-31.

[53] Majumder M, Ghosh AK, Steele R, Zhou XY, Phillips NJ, Ray R, Ray RB. Hepatitis C virus NS5A protein impairs TNF-mediated hepatic apoptosis, but not by an anti-Fas antibody, in transgenic mice. *Virology.* 2002 Mar 1; 294 (1): 94-105.

[54] Wang J, Tong W, Zhang X, Chen L, Yi Z, Pan T, Hu Y, Xiang L, Yuan Z. Hepatitis C virus non-structural protein NS5A interacts with FKBP38 and inhibits apoptosis in Huh7 hepatoma cells. *FEBS Lett.* 2006 Aug 7; 580 (18): 4392-400.

[55] Ciccaglione AR, Marcantonio C, Tritarelli E, Equestre M, Magurano F, Costantino A, Nicoletti L, Rapicetta M. The transmembrane domain of hepatitis C virus E1 glycoprotein induces cell death. *Virus Res.* 2004 Aug; 104 (1): 1-9.

[56] Chiou HL, Hsieh YS, Hsieh MR, Chen TY. HCV E2 may induce apoptosis of Huh-7 cells via a mitochondrial-related caspase pathway. *Biochem Biophys Res Commun.* 2006 Jun 23; 345 (1): 453-8.

[57] Schluger LK, Sheiner PA, Thung SN, Lau JY, Min A, Wolf DC, Fiel I, Zhang D, Gerber MA, Miller CM, Bodenheimer HC Jr. Severe recurrent cholestatic hepatitis C following orthotopic liver transplantation. *Hepatology* 1996 May; 23 (5): 971-6.

[58] Bernard PH, Le Bail B, Rullier A, Trimoulet P, Neau-Cransac M, Balabaud C, Bioulac-Sage P. Recurrence and accelerated progression of hepatitis C following liver transplantation. *Semin Liver Dis* 2000; 20 (4): 533-8.

[59] Doughty AL, Painter DM, McCaughan GW. Post-transplant quasispecies pattern remains stable over time in patients with recurrent cholestatic hepatitis due to hepatitis C virus. *J Hepatol* 2000 Jan; 32 (1): 126-34.

[60] Pessoa MG, Bzowej N, Berenguer M, Phung Y, Kim M, Ferrell L, Hassoba H, Wright TL. Evolution of hepatitis C virus quasispecies in patients with severe cholestatic hepatitis after liver transplantation. *Hepatology* 1999 Dec; 30 (6):1513-20.

[61]   Morales JM. Hepatitis C and renal transplantation: outcome of patients. *Nephrol Dial Transplant* 1995; 10 Suppl 6: 125-8.

[62]   Morales JM, Prieto C, Colina F, Andres A, Moreno F, Rodicio JL. Does cyclosporine induce clinical remission of dialysis – acquired active chronic hepatitis? *Nephron* 1989; 51 (1): 146-7.

[63]   Bloom RD, Lake JR. Emerging issues in hepatitis C virus-positive liver and kidney transplant recipients. *Am J Transplant* 2006 Oct; 6 (10): 2232–7.

[64]   Fabrizi F, Bromberg J, Elli A, Dixit V, Martin P. Review article: Hepatitis C virus and calcineurin inhibition after renal transplantation. *Aliment Pharmacol Ther* 2005 Oct; 22 (8): 657–66.

[65]   Fagiuoli S, Bruni F, Bravi M, Candusso M, Gaffuri G, Colledan M, Torre G. Cyclosporin in steroid-resistant autoimmune hepatitis and HCV-related liver diseases. *Dig Liver Dis* 2007 Nov; 39 Suppl 3: S379–85.

[66]   Nanmoku K, Imaizumi R, Tojimbara T, Nakajima I, Fuchinoue S, Sakamoto N, Watanabe M, Teraoka S. Effects of immunosuppressants on the progression of hepatitis C in hepatitis C virus-positive renal transplantation and the usefulness of interferon therapy. *Transplant Proc.* 2008 Sep; 40(7):2382-5.

[67]   Fernandes F, Poole DS, Hoover S, Middleton R, Andrei AC, Gerstner J, Striker R. Sensitivity of hepatitis C virus to cyclosporine A depends on nonstructural proteins NS5A and NS5B. *Hepatology* 2007 Oct; 46 (4): 1026–33.

[68]   Rostaing L, Izopet J, Sandres K, Cisterne JM, Puel J, Durand D. Changes in hepatitis C virus RNA viremia concentrations in long-term renal transplant patients after introduction of mycophenolate mofetil. *Transplantation.* 2000 Mar 15; 69(5):991-4.

[69]   Ramos-Casals M, Font J. Mycophenolate mofetil in patients with hepatitis C virus infection. *Lupus* 2005;14 Suppl 1: S64–S72.

[70]   Luan FL, Schaubel DE, Zhang H, Jia X, Pelletier SJ, Port FK, Magee JC, Sung RS. Impact of immunosuppressive regimen on survival of kidney transplant recipients with hepatitis C. *Transplantation.* 2008 Jun 15; 85(11):1601-6.

In: Hepatitis C Virus
Editors: A. P. Gonzales et al.

ISBN 978-1-61942-674-0
© 2012 Nova Science Publishers, Inc.

Chapter VII

Impact of Metabolic Factors on the Clinical Course of Patients with Hepatitis C Virus Infection

Hirokazu Takahashi and Toshihiko Mizuta
Department of Internal Medicine, Saga Medical School, Saga, Japan

ABSTRACT

It is well known that chronic hepatitis C virus (HCV) infection is the main cause of liver cirrhosis and hepatocellular carcinoma (HCC). In terms of the underlying mechanisms, many experimental and clinical studies have suggested that insulin resistance, oxidative stress, or subsequent abnormalglucose metabolism caused by obesity or HCV itself might play important roles in the progression of liver fibrosis and carcinogenesis. In this chapter, we discuss the associations between metabolic factors and the clinical course of HCV-infected patients.

IMPACT OF INSULIN RESISTANCE IN HCV INFECTION

It has been shown that HCV itself, including its core protein, directly induces insulin resistance by impairing the insulin-signaling pathway [1, 2]. It was also reported that insulin resistance is more severe in chronic HCV-infected patients than in patients with chronic hepatitis caused by another etiology [3]. Regardless of the relationship between insulin resistance and HCV infection, the possible effect of HCV on visceral fat accumulation remains unclear.

We have examined the relationship between insulin resistance and visceral fat accumulation in HCV-infected patients [4]. In that study, we compared the clinical characteristics of 87 chronic HCV-infected (CHC) patients with mild fibrosis (stage 1 or 2) with 125 sex- and age-matched patients with non-alcoholic fatty liver disease (NAFLD). Visceral fat area (VFA) at the umbilical level was measured by abdominal computed tomography (Figure 1) and divided into two grades: no visceral obesity (VFA <100 cm^2) and visceral obesity (VFA >100 cm^2). Insulin resistance was evaluated by the homeostasis model assessment of insulin resistance (HOMA-IR) and the quantitative insulin sensitivity check index (QUICKI), using the formulae HOMA-IR = fasting insulin (μU/ml) × fasting PG (mg/dl)/405 and QUICKI = 1/[log fasting insulin (μU/ml) ×log fasting PG (mg/dl)].Serum concentrations of soluble tumor necrosis factor-receptors(sTNFR)-1 and -2, and adiponectin were also measured.

Insulin resistance evaluated by HOMA-IR and QUICKI were both correlated with VFA (HOMA-IR: r=0.466. p<0.001; QUICKI: r=–0.449. p<0.001). HOMA-IR was higher in viscerally obese CHC patients than in viscerally obese NAFLD patients (2.9 ± 1.2 vs. 2.4 ± 1.5, p=0.048). Serum sTNFR-1 and -2 concentrations were also higher in CHC patients than in NAFLD patients with visceral obesity (sTNFR-1: 1.47 ± 0.64 ng/ml vs. 1.22 ± 0.28 ng/ml, p=0.028; sTNFR-2, 3.32 ± 0.89 ng/ml vs. 2.35 ± 0.69 ng/ml, p<0.001). In multivariate regression analysis, visceral obesity (VFA >100 cm^2) was independently associated with insulin resistance (odds ratio 7.85, p=0.015).

We found that increasing visceral fat accumulation was independently and significantly associated with the development of insulin resistance in CHC patients. Furthermore, pancreatic β cell function evaluated by HOMA-β was higher in CHC patients than in NAFLD patients with or without visceral obesity. These findings suggest that HCV infection may affect glucose metabolism regardless of the extent of visceral obesity, and that marked visceral fat accumulation significantly worsens insulin resistance. In addition, the progression of insulin resistance as a result of increased TNF activity in viscerally obese HCV-infected patients may be enhanced by a decrease in adiponectin secretion. Taken together, these findings suggest that HCV infection is a risk factor for the development of insulin resistance, particularly in patients with visceral obesity.

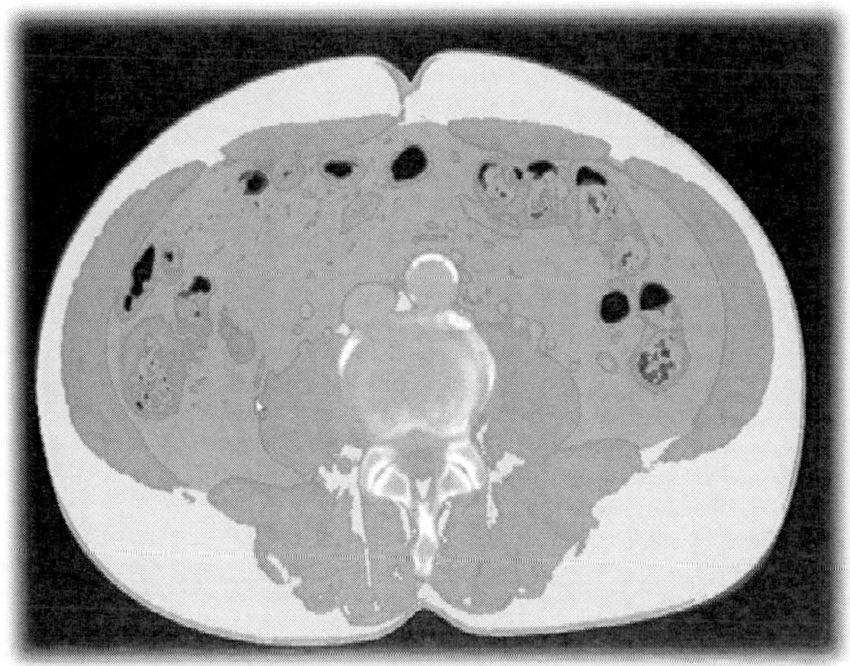

Figure 1. Visceral fat area was evaluated at umbilical level by computed tomography.

INSULIN RESISTANCE IS ASSOCIATED WITH THE SERUM ALANINE AMINOTRANSFERASE (ALT) LEVELS IN HCV INFECTION

Serum ALT activity is an important marker for the management of CHC patients [5] and for the diagnosis of liver diseases [6, 7], partly because it can be easily and repeatedly measured within clinical practice. Therefore, examining the associations between serum ALT levels with viral and host factors, including metabolic factors, would be useful to better understand the pathogenesis and natural course of CHC. Accordingly, we retrospectively examined the clinical, histological and virological characteristics of CHC patients to identify factors associated with serum ALT levels [8].

Table 1. Patients' characteristics stratified by serum ALT level

	ALT (IU/L)			p value
	<40	40-80	>80	
	n=58	n=83	n=59	
Age (yrs)	55.7±10.2	56.4±10.9	54.5±10.0	0.402[a]
Sex (male/female)	20/38	48/35	38/21	0.003[b]
Body weight (kg)	56.7±8.7	61.1±10.2	64.0±10.4	0.002[a]
Body mass index (kg/m^2)	22.8±2.4	23.9±3.0	24.2±3.2	0.017[a]
<22/22<	23/35	20/63	11/48	0.028[b]
<25/25<	48/10	54/29	40/19	0.061[b]
Alcohol consumption (g/day) (<20/20<)	48/10	64/19	42/17	0.142[b]
Glucose tolerance (NGT/IGT/DM)	42/13/3	45/30/8	35/17/7	0.231[b]
HCV RNA (KIU/ml)	2080.4±1595.2	1650.6±1395.6	1679.4±1586.8	0.171[a]
HCV genotype (1b/non-1b)	42/16	69/14	38/21	0.038[b]
Platelet (×10^3/mm^3)	184±63	153±56	149±48	0.002[a]
Fasting plasma glucose (mg/dl)	84.8±8.6	88.3±10.2	87.3±10.6	0.153[a]
Fasting plasma insulin (µU/ml)	7.06±3.99	9.17±4.43	12.53±7.17	<0.0001[a]
HOMA-IR	1.49±0.88	2.01±1.02	2.74±1.66	<0.0001[a]
Insulin sensitivity index (WBISI)	6.62±4.24	4.48±2.23	3.64±2.21	<0.0001[a]
Adiponectin (µg/ml)	11.9±5.9	10.4±4.6	9.9±4.4	0.426[a]
Leptin (ng/ml)				
Male	3.98±2.37	4.29±2.34	5.44±3.67	0.332[a]
Female	9.04±3.57	11.23±5.07	12.21±4.96	0.240[a]
Histological findings				
Grade of activity (A1/A2,A3)	35/20	17/59	15/42	<0.0001[a]
Stage of fibrosis (F1,F2/F3,F4)	51/4	53/23	41/16	0.005[b]
Grade of steatosis (<30%/>30%)	55/0	72/4	49/8	0.009[b]

a: Kruskal-Wallis test, b: χ^2 test.

In a retrospective analysis of 200 CHC patients who underwent liver biopsy, we classified the patients into three groups according to serum ALT levels as normal to minimal (<40 IU/l), mild (40–80 IU/l), and moderate to severe elevation (≥80 IU/l). All demographic and laboratory data were collected at the time of liver biopsy. All biopsies were evaluated for fibrosis, inflammation and steatosis. Glucose metabolism was assessed by various indices derived from oral glucose tolerance tests (OGTT), including HOMA-IR. We found that higher serum ALT levels were significantly associated with male sex, lower high-density lipoprotein cholesterol, higher HOMA-IR, and higher grades of histological inflammation and steatosis (Table 1). Serum ALT levels were positively correlated with HOMA-IR (r=0.297, p<0.001) (Figure 2). In multivariate logistic regression analysis, male sex (odds ratio 3.59, p=0.001), HOMA-IR >2 (odds ratio 3.12, p=0.017) and pathological fibrosis stage F3-4 (odds ratio 3.31, p=0.048) were independently associated with serum ALT ≥40 IU/l. We concluded from these results that insulin resistance is a significant risk factor for ALT elevations, and that insulin resistance might offer a new target to correct ALT elevations.

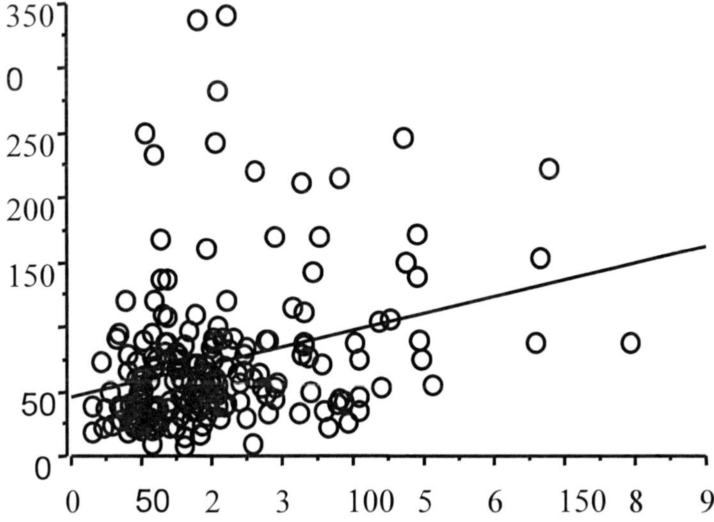

Figure 2. Correlation between serum ALT levels and HOMA-IR. Serum ALT levels were positively correlated with HOMA-IR (r=0.297, p<0.001 by Pearson's correlation coefficient and Fisher's test).

ASSOCIATIONS BETWEEN THE EFFICACY OF ANTI-VIRAL THERAPY AND INSULIN RESISTANCE IN CHC PATIENTS

Peg-interferon (PEG) plus ribavirin (RBV) therapy is widely accepted as the gold standard therapy for CHC. About 60% of patients achieve a sustained virological response (SVR) to the therapy. However, the factors that contribute to the efficacy of this therapy are unclear. One study reported that host-related factors, including obesity-associated hepatic steatosis and insulin resistance, influenced the efficacy of PEG/RBV therapy [9, 10]. HOMA-IR is thought to represent hepatic insulin resistance because it is calculated from fasting plasma glucose and insulin levels. Matsuda and DeFronzo [11] reported a method to estimate the whole-body insulin sensitivity index (WBISI) via a simple OGTT. Therefore, we examined whether these metabolic factors influenced the anti-viral effect of PEG/RBV therapy [12].

Fifty-one patients with genotype 1b and a high viral load who received PEG/RBV therapy for 48 weeks were included in the study. HOMA-IR and WBISI calculated from 75-g OGTTs and serum levels of sTNFR-2were determined before therapy. Patients who achieved SVR had significantly lower HOMA-IR and sTNFR-2 levels and a higher WBISI compared with patients who did not achieve SVR (Table 2). The positive predictive value for SVR was 0.653 for HOMA-IR <2 and 0.846 for WBISI ≥6. Thus, WBISI may be a highly specific predictor for SVR in PEG/RBV therapy.

Next, to investigate whether eradication of HCV by interferon (IFN) therapy influences systemic glucose metabolism, we analyzed the changes in OGTT-determined indices, includingHOMA-IR, HOMA-β, insulinogenic index (II), WBISI, and area under the curves for plasma glucose (AUC_{PG}) and serum insulin (AUC_{SI}),which were determined before and after 6 months of IFN therapy in 72CHC (48 patients with SVR and 24 patients without SVRs) [13]. The serum levels of sTNFR-2 were measured in 28 patients with SVR and 16 patients without SVRs. Among patients who achieved SVR, HOMA-β (p=0.0004) and AUC_{SI} (p=0.002) were significantly decreased and WBISI was increased (p=0.009), compared with patients without SVR, although there were no significant changes in HOMA-IR, II or AUC_{PG} (Table 3). Serum sTNFR-2 levels decreased significantly after therapy in patients who achieved SVR (p=0.001). By comparison, there were no changes in any of these indices in patients without SVR. Overall, these findings suggest that eradication of HCV by IFN therapy could improve whole-body insulin resistance and insulin hypersecretion, as well as reduce serum TNFα levels.

Table 2. Differences in characteristics between the sustained and non-sustained virological responders

	Sustained responders (n = 23)	Non-sustained responders (n = 28)	P
Age (years)	52.2 ± 11.7	56.8 ± 7.6	0.19
Male (%)	16 (69.6)	16 (57.1)	0.40
Weight (kg)	59.1 ± 8.5	60.6 ± 10.4	0.72
BMI (kg/m^2)	23.0 ± 3.3	23.4 ± 2.8	0.42
AST (IU/l)	45.7 ± 18.1	71.1 ± 41.1	0.02
ALT (IU/l)	58.8 ± 32.5	84.0 ± 52.7	0.08
HCV viral load (kIU/ml)	2,102.6 ± 1628.2	2,255.4 ± 1358.1	0.51
Histological findings (n = 47)			
Necroinflammation (A1/A2 + A3)	9/10	5/23	0.05
Fibrosis (F1 + F2/F3 + F4)	17/2	19/9	0.16
Steatosis (<33%/>33%)	19/0	25/3	0.26
HOMA-IR	1.56 ± 0.96	2.67 ± 1.61	0.003
HOMA-β	120.2 ± 69.4	204.9 ± 144.9	0.01
Insulinogenic index	0.98 ± 0.96	1.18 ± 1.25	0.60
WBISI	6.44 ± 4.63	3.87 ± 2.95	0.004
sTNFR2 (pg/ml)	2,612.4 ± 714.5	3,206.3 ± 768.8	0.004

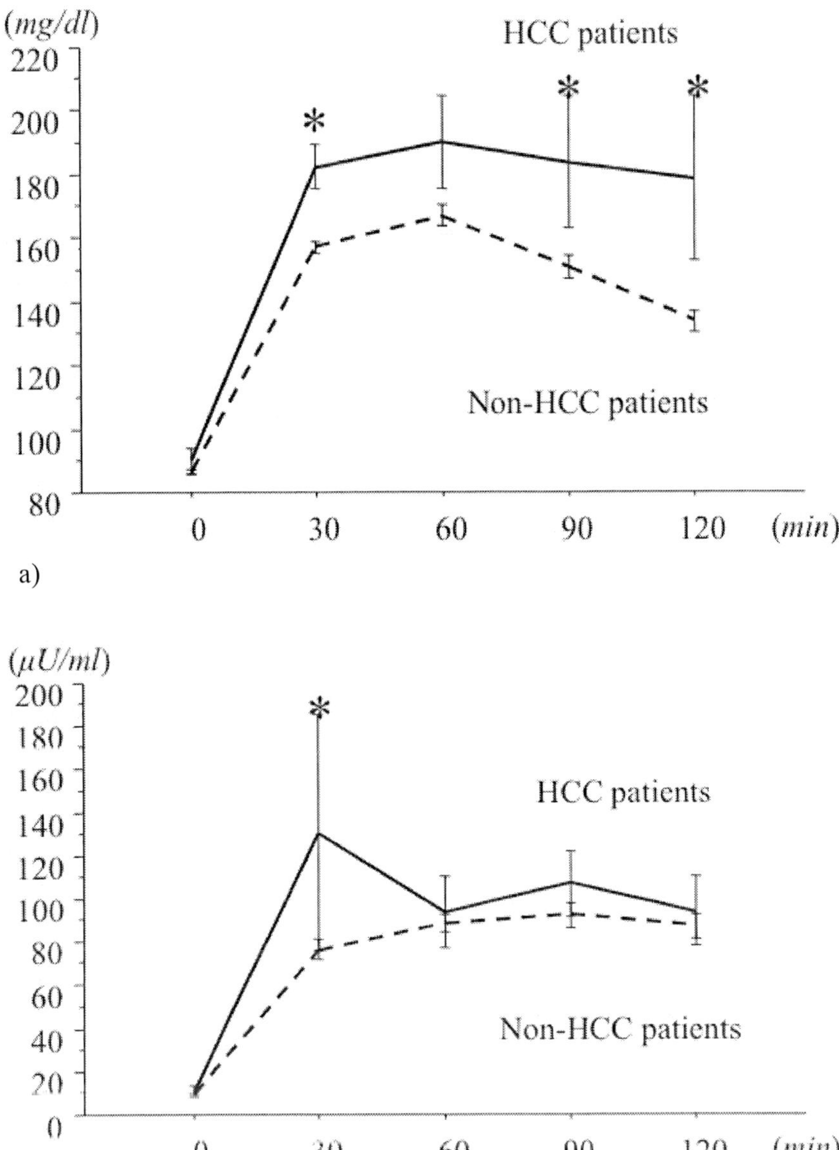

Figure 3. a) Serum glucose levels and b) insulin levels on 75-gOGTT. Thick line patients who developed HCC. Thin line patients without HCC. *P < 0.05 by Mann–Whitney U test. Error bar ± standard deviation.

**Table 3. Changes in variables before and 6 months
after interferon therapy in sustained responders
(n = 48)*sTNFR2 was analyzed in 28 subjects**

	Before	After	p value
Body mass index (kg/m2)	23.3±3.2	23.0±3.2	0.098
HOMA-β	174±211	105±60	<0.001
HOMA-IR	1.86±1.08	1.67±0.93	0.566
Insulinogenic index	1.06±1.01	0.92±1.18	0.361
WBISI	5.03±2.45	6.24±3.79	0.009
PG-AUC	169±39	162±36	0.100
SI-AUC	83±49	64±38	0.002
sTNFR2 (pg/ml)*	2682±759	2408±628	0.001

HEPATOCARCINOGENESIS AND GLUCOSE INTOLERANCE IN CHC PATIENTS

Several recent epidemiological studies have shown that diabetes mellitus (DM) is a risk factor for HCC in CHC patients [14, 15], although studies in Taiwan revealed no such association [16, 17]. Thus, it is still unclear whether DM is a clinically significant risk factor for HCC. Therefore, we did a study to determine the association between DM/post-challenge hyperglycemia and hepatocarcinogenesis in CHC patients [18]. A total of 203 CHC patients (108 males, mean age 54.3 ± 10.8 years; 95 females, mean age 56.6 ± 10.3 years; genotype 1b/2a/2b/3a: 152/38/12/1) who underwent liver biopsy and a 75-g OGTT, and who were treated with IFN, were enrolled in this study. None of the subjects had been treated with anti-diabetic drugs. The subjects underwent ultrasonography and/or computed tomography every 6 months after completing IFN therapy. Thirteen patients, including one patient who achieved SVR with IFN, developed HCC.

Among patients who developed HCC (HCC group), the glucose levels at 30 (p=0.002), 90 (p=0.033) and 120 (p=0.001) min, and the insulin levels at 30 min (p=0.017) during the OGTT were significantly higher than those in patients without HCC (non-HCC group) (Figure 3a,b). There were no significant differences in fasting glucose or insulin levels between the two groups. The cumulative HCC occurrence rates among patients with 120-min post-challenge glucose levels of >200 mg/dl and those with levels of <200 mg/dl are shown in Figure 4a. While the HCC occurrence rates at 3 and 5 years were 3.3% and 4.3% in patients with 120-min glucose <200 mg/dl, the corresponding rates were 15.0% and 28.1% in patients with 120-min glucose >200 mg/dl. There was a significant difference in the HCC occurrence rate between patients with 120-min glucose <200 mg/dl versus those with >200 mg/dl ($p<0.001$). Figure 4b shows the cumulative HCC occurrence rates in patients with a liver steatosis area of >5% and those with a liver steatosis area of <5%. The rates at 3 and 5 years were 14.3% and 20.4% in patients with a liver steatosis area of >5% versus 2.9% and 4.7%, respectively, in patients with a liver steatosis area of <5%. There was a significant difference in the HCC occurrence rate between patients with a liver steatosis area of >5% versus those with a liver steatosis area of <5% ($p<0.001$). In multivariate analysis, male sex, age >65 years, excessive alcohol consumption, non-SVR, liver steatosis area >5% in liver specimens, and 120-min post-challenge hyperglycemia were risk factors for the development of HCC. After matching subjects for sex, age, alcohol intake and response to the IFN therapy, advanced fibrosis stages [hazard ratio (HR) 2.8], liver steatosis (HR 5.4) and 120-min post-challenge hyperglycemia (HR 4.9) were significant risk factors for the development of HCC. Furthermore, after matching for fibrosis stage, liver steatosis (HR 5.7) and 120-min post-challenge hyperglycemia (HR 6.9) remained as significant factors for HCC development. We conclude from these findings that post-challenge hyperglycemia is an independent risk factor for HCC in CHC patients.

CONCLUSIONS

Metabolic factors including visceral obesity, hepatic or whole-body insulin resistance, and post-challenge hyperglycemia have a negative influence on every aspect of the clinical course in HCV-infected patients. Therapeutic interventions that target these metabolic factors, including lifestyle modifications or pharmacotherapy with insulin sensitizers, for example, could improve the prognosis of CHC patients.

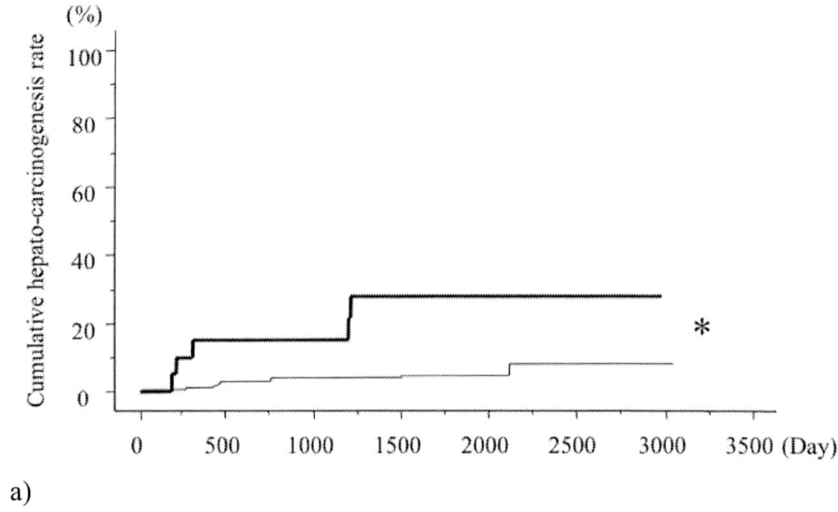

a)

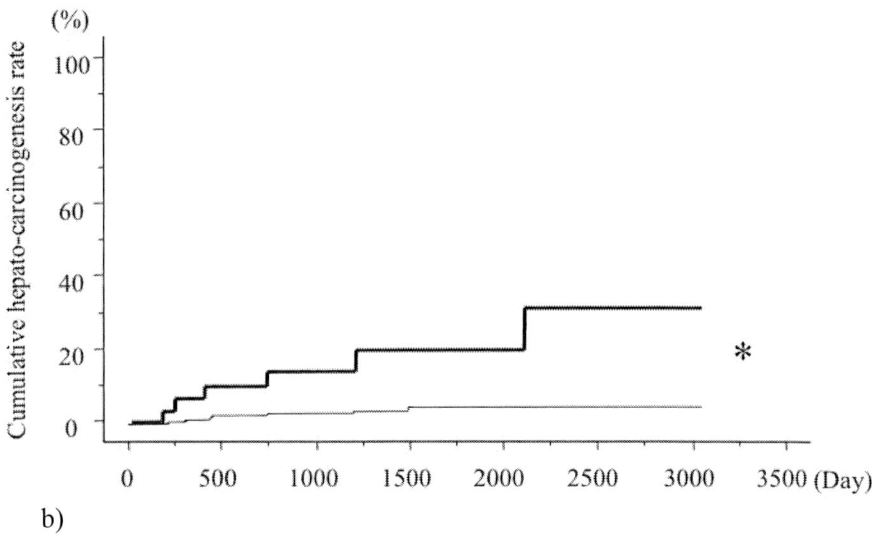

b)

Figure 4. a) The cumulative HCC occurrence rates in patients with 120 min post-challenge hyperglycemia (serum glucose level more than 200 mg/dl at 120 min on 75-g OGTT; thick line) and patients without hyperglycemia (serum glucose level less than 200 mg/dl at 20 min on 75-g OGTT; thin line). b) The cumulative HCC occurrence rates in patients with liver steatosis of more than 5% (thick line) and patients with liver steatosis of 5% or less (thin line). *P < 0.001 by log-rank test.

REFERENCES

[1] Shintani Y, Fujie H, Miyoshi H, Tsutsumi T, Tsukamoto K, Kimura S, et al. Hepatitis C virus infection and diabetes: direct involvement of the virus in the development of insulin resistance. *Gastroenterology.* 2004;126:840–848.

[2] Kawaguchi T, Yoshida T, Harada M, Hisamoto T, Nagao Y, Ide T, et al. Hepatitis C virus down-regulates insulin receptor sub- strates 1 and 2 through up-regulation of suppressor of cytokine signaling 3. *Am J Pathol.* 2004;165:1499–508.

[3] Persico M, Masarone M, La Mura V, Persico E, Moschella F, Svelto M, et al. Clinical expression of insulin resistance in hep- atitis C and B virus-related chronic hepatitis: differences and similarities. *World J Gastroenterol.* 2009;15:462–466.

[4] Eguchi Y, Mizuta T, Ishibashi E, Kitajima Y, Oza N, Nakashita S, et al. Hepatitis C virus infection enhances insulin resistance induced by visceral fat accumulation. *Liver Int.* 2009;29:213–220.

[5] Alberti A. Towards more individualized management of hepatitis C virus patients with initially or persistently normal alanine aminotransferase levels. *J Hepatol.* 2005;42:266–274.

[6] Pratt DS, Kaplan MM. Evaluation of abnormal liver-enzyme results in asymptomatic patients. *N Engl J Med.* 2000;342: 1266 1271.

[7] Crax`ı A, Almasio P. Diagnostic approach to liver enzyme ele- vation. *J Hepatol.* 1996;25(Suppl 1):47–51.

[8] Kobayashi Y, Kawaguchi Y, Mizuta T, Kuwashiro T, Oeda S, Oza N, et al.Metabolic factors are associated with serum alanine aminotransferase levels in patients with chronic hepatitis C.*J Gastroenterol.* 2011;46:529-535.

[9] Charlton MR, Pockros P, Harrison SA. Impact of obesity on treatment of chronic hepatitis C. *Hepatology.* 2006;43:1177–1186.

[10] Harrison SA. Insulin resistance among patients with chronic hepatitis C: etiology and impact on treatment. *ClinGastroenterolHepatol.* 2008;6:864–876.

[11] Matsuda M, DeFronzo R. Insulin sensitivity indices obtained from oral glucose tolerance testing: comparison with the eugly- cemic insulin clamp. *Diabetes Care.* 1999;22:1462–1470.

[12] Mizuta T, Kawaguchi Y, EguchiY, Takahashi H, ArioK, Akiyama T, et al. Whole-Body Insulin Sensitivity Index Is a Highly Specific Predictive Marker for Virological Response to Peginterferon Plus Ribavirin Therapy in Chronic Hepatitis C Patients with Genotype 1b and High Viral Load. *Dig Dis Sci* (2010) 55:183–189.

[13] Kawaguchi Y, Mizuta T, Oza N, Takahashi H, Ario K, Yoshimura T, et al. Eradication of hepatitis C virus by interferon improves whole-body insulin resistance and hyperinsulinaemia in patients with chronic hepatitis C.*Liver Int.* 2009;29:871-877.

[14] Veldt BJ, Chen W, Heathcote EJ, Wedemeyer H, Reichen J, Hofmann WP, et al. Increased risk of hepatocellular carcinoma among patients with hepatitis C cirrhosis and diabetes mellitus. *Hepatology.* 2008;47:1856–1862.

[15] Chen CL, Yang HI, Yang WS, Liu CJ, Chen PJ, You SL, et al. Metabolic factors and risk of hepatocellular carcinoma by chronichepatitis B/C infection: a follow-up study in Taiwan. *Gastroenterology.* 2008;135:111–121.

[16] Tung HD, Wang JH, Tseng PL, Hung CH, Kee KM, Chen CH, et al. Neither diabetes mellitus nor overweight is a risk factor for hepatocellular carcinoma in a dual HBV and HCV endemic area: community cross-sectional and case–control studies. *Am J Gastroenterol.* 2010;105:624–631.

[17] Lai MS, Hsieh MS, Chiu YH, Chen TH. Type 2 diabetes and hepatocellular carcinoma: a cohort study in high prevalence area of hepatitis virus infection. *Hepatology.* 2006;43:1295–1302.

[18] Takahashi H, Mizuta T, Eguchi Y, Kawaguchi Y, Kuwashiro T, OedaS,et al.Post-challenge hyperglycemia is a significant risk factor for the development of hepatocellular carcinoma in patients with chronic hepatitis C.*J Gastroenterol.* 2011;46:790-798.

Index

I

J